FSMA Compliant in One Week

Be the FSMA Expert in Your Organization

Rob Kooijmans
Kitty Appels

Published by Best Seller Publishing®, Pasadena, CA
Best Seller Publishing® is a registered trademark
Printed in the United States of America.
ISBN: 978-1-949535-17-4

Most Best Seller Publishing® titles are available at special quantity discounts for bulk purchases for sales promotions, premiums, fundraising, and educational use. Special versions or book excerpts can also be created to fit specific needs.

For more information, please write:
Best Seller Publishing®
1346 Walnut Street, #205
Pasadena, CA 91106
or call 1(626) 765 9750
Toll Free: 1(844) 850-3500
Visit us online at: www.BestSellerPublishing.org

Contents

Introduction 1

Chapter 1
Introduction 5

Chapter 2
FSMA Overview and Timing 21

Chapter 3
Creating Your Implementation Plan 51

Chapter 4
Preventive Controls for Human and Animal Food 55

Chapter 5
Implementation Plan Preventive Controls for
Human and Animal Food 91

Chapter 6
The Supply Chain Program and the Foreign
Supplier Verification Program 95

Chapter 7
Implementation Plan Supplier Management,
FSVP and VQIP 115

Chapter 8
Intentional Adulteration and Food Defense 119

Chapter 9
Implementation Plan Intentional Adulteration
and Food Defense 137

Chapter 10
Sanitary Transportation of Human
and Animal Food 141

Chapter 11
Implementation Plan Sanitary Transport....................149

Chapter 12
The Produce Safety and Sprout Safety Rules..............153

Chapter 13
Implementation Plan Pro-duce Safety
and Sprout Safety...183

Chapter 14
Training for FSMA Compliance..................................187

About the Authors 197

Introduction

The Food Safety Modernization Act in the United States of America (or in short FSMA) has been the biggest change in food safety legislation in decades. And not only in the USA! This framework of several rule has a global impact as all food producing companies exporting food stuff to the USA are impacted by FSMA as well.

We have been following the creation of FSMA over several years as from the onset it was clear that this new legislation would have a major impact. By the same token we have helped many companies to successfully become complaint to the various rules within FSMA over the last couple of years.

Naturally, the US FDA has created formal training on various parts of FSMA. While this training does result in a certified, qualified individual status for the students, it does not give a hands-on structure for implementing all the requirements of FSMA. Nor does the formal training dive into the level of detail at which processes must be defined. A large part of FSMA does leave room for interpretation and with the right information companies can come to an effective and efficient implementation of all the requirements.

This book is not just going to cover a lot of boring theory or just the legal requirements. No – this book is hands-on and will deliver the information to you in a very clear and understandable format. Next to this you will get easy to implement tools which are included as downloads via QR codes throughout the book. Every second chapter of this book (except for the introduction of course) is followed by a so-called "working chapter". In these chapters you will find guidance on the actions you need to take to get FSMA compliant in your company.

An important thing to note here is that even for a Qualified Individual, receiving formal, FDA certified training is not a mandatory requirement in FSMA. Any Qualified Individual can be qualified by a combination of education, training and experience. As longs a you properly document this you are OK. That's why you will get a certificate at completion of the FSMA Masterclass. And you can use this together with any other training, education or experiences to prove that you are a Qualified Individual in relation to FSMA.

So instead of spending at least two days per relevant FSMA rule in a boring classroom training and getting little to no guidance on how to implement things – you can now learn all you need to know, create your own implementation plan in the working chapters and get easy to implement tools from this book.

We are sure this book is going to be a strong starting point for FSMA compliance in your company. For those of you who wish to have even more guidance, we also have an online FSMA Masterclass and we even host a combined FSMA Masterclass / PCQI Training (with official FDA approved certificate) both in the USA and in Europe. For more information have a look at our website: https://foodsafety-university.thinkific.com/courses/fsma-masterclass

Together we continue to improve food safety everywhere.
Rob Kooijmans & Kitty Appels
Food Safety Experts

CHAPTER 1

Introduction

I. WHY THIS BOOK

*T*he *FDA Food Safety Modernization Act to amend the Federal Food, Drug, and Cosmetic Act with respect to the safety of the food supply* (or in short FSMA) has been the biggest change in food safety legislation in decades, and not only in the US.

We have been following the creation of FSMA over several years. From the onset, it was clear that its framework would also have a major impact on all companies producing and exporting foodstuff to the US. By the same token, since FSMA has been introduced, we have helped many companies to successfully become compliant with its various rules.

Naturally, the US FDA has created formal training on various parts of FSMA. While this training does result in a certified, "Qualified Individual" status for the students, it does not give a hands-on structure for implementing all of the requirements of FSMA. Nor does the formal training dive into the level of detail at which processes must be defined. A large part of FSMA leaves room for interpretation, and with the right information, companies can achieve an effective and efficient implementation of all of the requirements.

This book is not just going to cover a lot of boring theory or legal requirements. No – this book is hands-on and will deliver the information to you in a very clear and understandable format. In addition to this, you will get easy-to-implement tools, which are included as downloads via QR codes throughout the book. Every second chapter of this book (the introduction) is followed by a "working chapter". In these chapters you will find guidance on the actions you need to take to become FSMA-compliant within your company.

We are sure this book is going to be a strong starting point for FSMA compliance in your company. For those of you who wish to receive further guidance, we also have an online FSMA Masterclass and we even host a combined FSMA Masterclass / PCQI Training (with official FDA-approved certificate) both in the US and in Europe.

An important thing to note here is that even for a Qualified Individual, receiving formal FDA-certified training is not a mandatory requirement in FSMA. Any Qualified Individual can be qualified by a combination of education, training and experience. As longs a you properly document this, you are OK. That is why you will get a certificate upon completion of the FSMA Masterclass. And you can use thisalongside any other training, education or experiences to prove that you are a Qualified Individual in relation to FSMA.

So instead of spending at least two days on each FSMA rule in a boring classroom training setting and getting little to no guidance on how to implement things – you can now learn all you need to know, create your own implementation plan in the working chapters and get practical tools from this book.

For more information on our online FSMA Masterclass, have a look at our website: https://foodsafety-university. thinkific.com/courses/fsma-masterclass

We hope this book provides you with the insights and information you need to come to an effective implementation of all the relevant aspects of FSMA in your organization.

Together we continue to improve food safety everywhere.

Rob Kooijmans & Kitty Appels
Food Safety Experts

II. HOW AND WHY FSMA CAME TO BE

After almost two years in the making, FSMA was signed by President Obama in January 2011. An early version, called the Food Safety Enhancement Act, was approved by the House of Representatives in 2009; then, at the end of 2010, the US Senate approved a revised version under the name of the Food Safety Modernization Act as an amendment of the existing law, the Federal Food, Drug and Cosmetic Act (FFDCA) of 1938.

FSMA's sheer complexity made its implementation quite slow. Public comments on proposed rules opened in 2013, and the first set of final rules were published in 2015. As of today (September 2018), FSMA has been implemented almost in its entirety.

When US Congress chose the word "modernization" instead of "enhancement", it was not simply trying to find a synonym. The previous 1938 law came from a world that no longer existed, so a simple enhancement clearly would not be enough. An upgrade to modern times was necessary.

When lawmakers started to work on a modern food safety law, there were many signs that the food system was getting out of control, and a drastic change was necessary.

Too many people were dying or falling ill due to food poisoning.

While the US Congress was discussing the Food Safety Enhancement Act in 2009, the country was experiencing one of the most serious foodborne illness incidents in the recent years: the Peanut Corporation of America (PCA) *Salmonella* outbreak.

PCA was a peanut-processing business, which sold both raw and processed peanuts. In 2006, when a lab test found Salmonella in their products, the company management did not stop sales or warn customers or the authorities. Instead, they kept on doing more tests until they got negative results they could show, and even got to the point of faking sanitary certificates.

Unsurprisingly, a serious *Salmonella* outbreak followed, which caused nine deaths, while at least 714 people in 47 states fell ill and were hospitalised (half of them were children). The company's owner Stewart Parnell was eventually convicted and sentenced to 28 years (the Federal authorities had recommended life imprisonment) and the company went bankrupt.

The PCA case is an extreme example of large-scale profit-driven food poisoning.

In most cases however, serious foodborne illnesses are unintentional. In 2006 for example, water contaminated with animal faeces likely caused an E. coli outbreak in fresh spinach, which killed 3 people and sickened at least 276.

The PCA and E. coli cases above were not serious incidents in an otherwise healthy food system. Rather, they were the tip of the iceberg of many food safety incidents that were killing thousands of people every year. Data published by CDC (the Centre for Disease Control and Prevention) in 2011 estimated that "each year roughly 1 in 6 Americans (or 48 million people) gets sick, 128,000 are hospitalized, and 3,000 die of foodborne diseases." That data is often used as an introduction to FSMA. The same report however, has a much more worrying part: 56% of those deaths were caused by "unspecified agents transmitted through food." Poisoned food was killing people, but in most cases no one knew exactly how.

Food safety incidents are also a significant cost for the healthcare system. A 2015 study by Ohio State University, estimated that the average national cost of foodborne illness is between $55.5 billion $93.2 billion

Data provided by HorizonScan gives a more detailed picture of the state of food safety in the US in the last ten years. From 2008 to 2017, there were 6,836 reported food safety incidents, which were caused by 111 different types of contaminations. Five of them were responsible for 80% of total incidents:

- Aflatoxins
- Listeria
- Salmonella
- Unauthorised additives
- Undeclared allergens

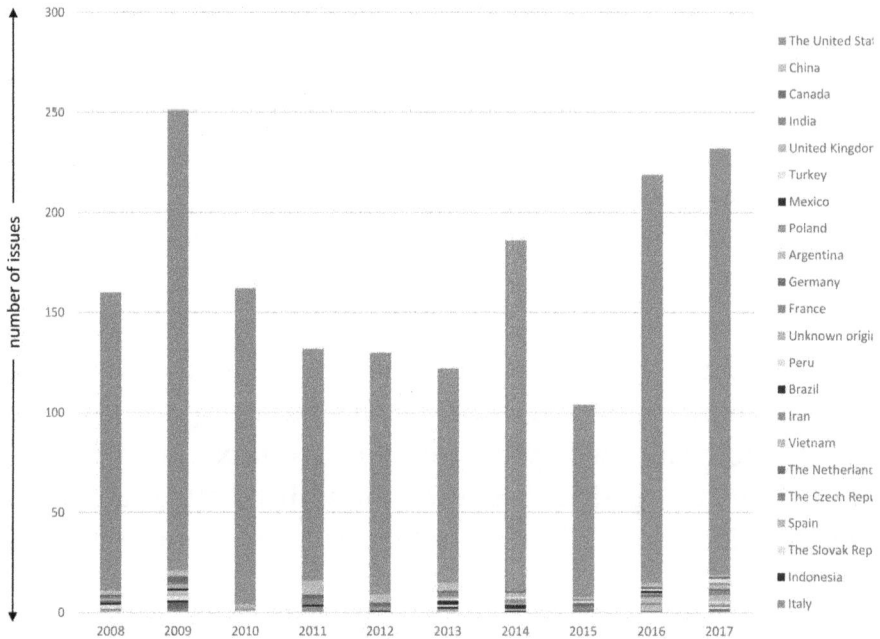

Total number of USA related food safety issues by country of origin.

As we can see from the chart above with data from HorizonScan, the progression of food incidents in the USA is not linear from year to year. The trend, however, is undoubtedly upward. A higher number of incidents does not necessarily mean that the food protection system has gotten worse. In fact, it can also mean that it is more capable of detecting food safety issues.

Food recalls cost the food industry millions of dollars every year.

Food safety incidents have a high social cost but are also a financial issue for the food industry. A product recall is both a sanitary and a PR crisis with repercussions at many levels: the cost of the recall itself, lost sales, damaged reputation, etc.

Comprehensive and updated data on the financial burden of food recalls is scarce, but   there are two recent studies we can quote.

An analysis of more than 100,000 insurance industry claims for product recalls by Allianz Global Corporate & Specialty. Key findings:

- The F&B sector is the second most affected by food recalls
- The average claim value is €1.31m
- The average claim value for a large recall is €7.92m

A 2011 report by the Grocery Manufacturers Association, based on a survey with 36 members. Key findings:

- 81% of respondents deem financial risk from recalls as significant to catastrophic
- 58% have been affected by a product recall event in the last five years
- 77% of them experienced recalls that had a financial impact of up to $30 million.

For large food companies, the financial impact of food recalls can be much higher than $30 million. Two notable examples are the Maggi instant noodle recall in India, which cost Nestle half-billion dollars and a milk recall which cost New Zealand's milk giant Fonterra over €100 million.

These cases are also important cautionary tales, and for two reasons. First: they prove that they can happen even to companies with the highest budgets to spend on food safety standards. Second: both recalls were precautionary, meaning they were issued over a *potential* food safety risk. Eventually, there were no consequences on public health and while this is certainly a positive outcome, it makes food safety an even greater liability for food companies.

Keeping track of food origins was becoming more and more difficult.

Food safety incidents are unfortunate events, but they could also serve as case studies for health authorities and food companies to make sure they do not happen again. Unfortunately, a globalised and incredibly complex food supply chain is making that task very difficult.

A good example of this is a 2016 Salmonella outbreak linked to hot peppers imported from Mexico and sold to restaurants.

In the investigation that followed, the CDC tried to find out exactly at what point between the farms and the restaurants the hot peppers were contaminated. However, the intricate web of intermediaries in the farm-to-table journey of the contaminated food – pictured below - made that search unsuccessful.

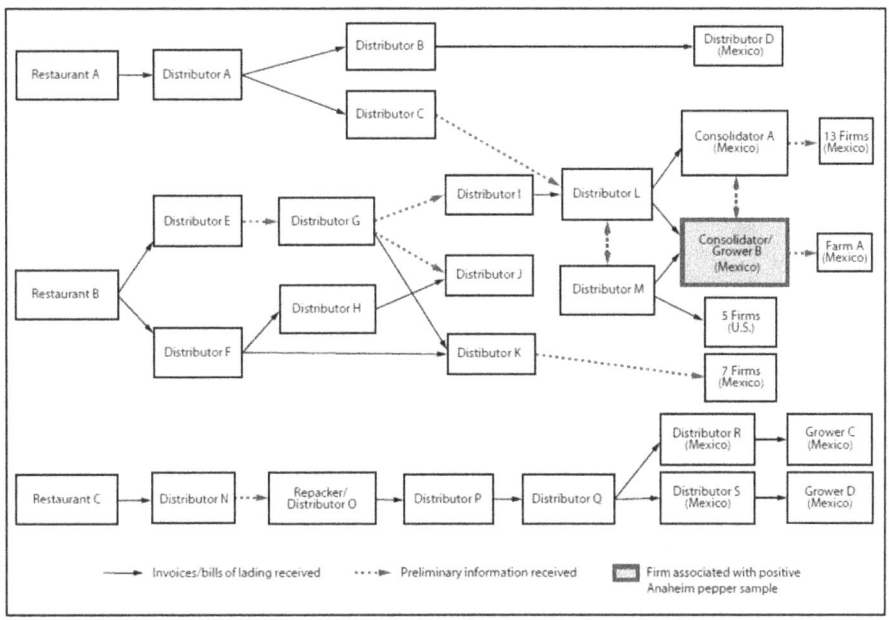

The chart above illustrates what can happen when a contaminated ingredient is at least identified. With processed multi-ingredient foods, things can get even more complicated. During the investigations following the horsemeat scandal in 2013, the National Audit Office in the UK reported that a pizza was in fact made with 35 ingredients that passed through 60 different countries, although on the label its country of origin was Ireland.

It was therefore clear that in a system where food travels the world with multiple stops, FSMA had to focus also on the food coming from foreign suppliers, not only on the domestic side.

Indeed, that shift in focus started to show some positive effects. Available data from HorizonScan as shown in the chart below, indicates that the situation improved in terms of the FDA consistently being the first food safety authority to pick up more food safety issues over the last years.

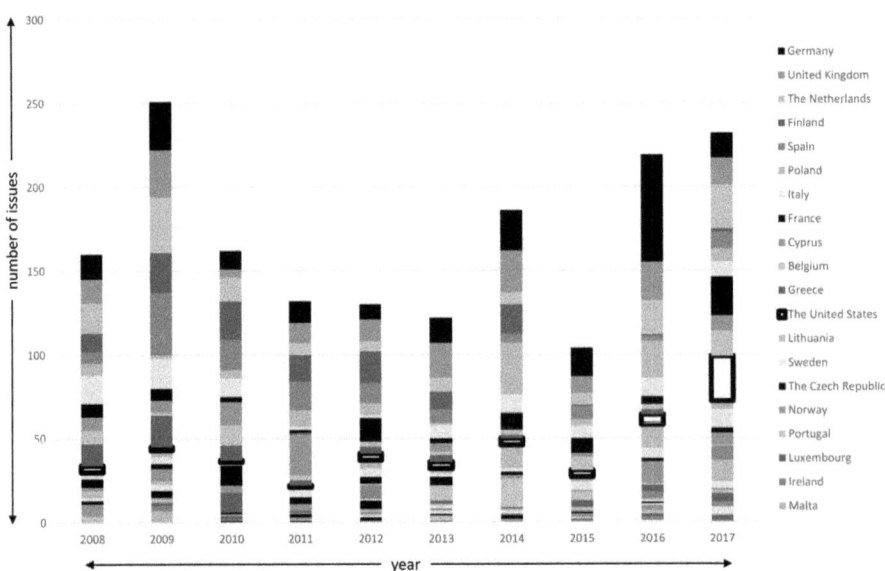

Total number of USA related food safety issues notified by various counties

Consumers were losing trust in food brands.

Finally, what made a new food safety law necessary was that consumers were losing trust in how genuinely food brands were trying to produce healthy food without unnecessary chemicals.

A survey conducted by Edelman in 2012 highlighted a growing concern in consumers about the sources of their food: 22% of respondents cited safety and production as one of the reasons why food production in America "is on the wrong track." 81% said they prefer US-grown foods, while 69% wanted to know where their food comes from.

III. THE PROTECTIVE NET OF FSMA

At its core, the purpose of FSMA is to cast a wider and tighter food protection net around consumers and the food industry in the US.

Food protection can take many forms. A useful way to represent it is the food risk matrix, which is divided into four quadrants: food fraud, food safety, food quality and food defence.

https://www.foodsafetystrategies.com/ext/resources/ FSS_Event/2017/2017_Presentations/Food-Fraud-and-Vulnerability-Assessment.pdf?1515701161

Food Quality	Food Fraud	Motivation Gain: Economic
Food Safety	Food Defence	Harm: Public Health, Economic, or Terror
Unintentional	Intentional	
Action		

Food fraud

A common definition of food fraud is the "deliberate and intentional substitution, addition, tampering, or misrepresentation of food, food ingredients, or food packaging; or false or misleading statements made about a product for economic gain."

The most important part in this definition is "economic gain." Because profit is the primary goal of food fraud, in most cases there is no eventual risk for public health.

The EU horsemeat scandal is an example of a large-scale food fraud where not a single person was reported sick. Also, food fraud is not limited to food adulteration, but includes conducts outside the food risk matrix, such as misbranding and theft.

However, food fraud *is* also a health risk, as the negligent conduct of the fraudster may unintentionally harm people. The 2008 melamine milk scandal in China, where six infants died and an estimated 54,000 were hospitalised, remains one of the worst examples of the unintentional consequences of food fraud. That incident was one of the lowest points in the history of food safety and a major turning point towards a tighter food protection system worldwide.

Food fraud is a very common crime around the world. What makes it so appealing to fraudsters is the opportunity to obtain maximum profit with minimum risk. The most targeted foods are also the most expensive ones. Here we will provide a few examples, although the list is by no means exhaustive.

Meat. In the above-mentioned 2013 horsemeat scandal, beef meat was mixed with considerable amounts of horse meat to lower its production cost and increase profits. The response of the authorities was tighter controls and the creation of the Food Fraud Network. That wouldn't be enough to stop fraudsters, though: still today, criminals are being arrested for the same type of fraud.

Olive oil. The adulteration of olive oil is almost as old as olive oil itself. Very frequent ways this is done is by selling further processed olive oil as extra virgin olive oil or mixing different oils without declaring it on the label.

Honey. According to a 2016 EU report, 14.2% of honey is likely to be adulterated. Again, the most expensive ones are a favourite target, like Manuka from New Zealand. In 2014, the leading Manuka association calculated that the consumption of Manuka honey in the UK alone exceeds the total production of New Zealand. That clearly means that a lot of honey that is sold as Manuka is not what consumers expect it to be.

Fish. Last year, a report from non-profit ocean conservation group Oceana revealed how "seafood swaps" is as a global practice. The typical example is Asian catfish, which is mislabelled and sold as eighteen different – and more expensive – types of fish.

Food fraud is a very pervasive crime and still very difficult to fight. Unfortunately, there's no comprehensive data on the phenomenon, because not all cases are discovered by authorities and food companies are not always keen on reporting that they were victims of food frauds.

Another survey-based report by the GMA from 2010 can help shed some light. Its conclusions are worrying: economic adulteration and counterfeiting cost the food industry between $10 and $15 billion per year globally. For a single company, being a victim of food fraud case may cost between 2% and 15% of annual revenues.

Food quality and food safety

While food safety and food quality are both unintentional acts, food quality issues do not necessarily result in food safety issues.

Food safety incidents can be caused by different things: physical contamination (plastic, stones, bones, etc), chemical contamination (pesticides, cleaning agents, etc.) and bacteria or allergens not declared on the packaging.

At a more general level, a food safety issue is also a food quality issue. In the context of the food risk matrix however, food quality has more to do with customers' expectations regarding the appearance and texture of food. A food processing operation that is not investing enough resources in equipment and quality control is more likely to incur food quality issues.

Food defence

Food defence is the protection against intentional food contamination whose specific purpose is to harm people.

Intentional food contamination can happen at different scales. On the small side of the spectrum, we find individual criminal acts, for example when a murderer kills someone by poisoning their food. The real concern of FSMA, however, is to prevent large-scale incidents like food terrorist attacks, industrial sabotage, or other acts with purely criminal intent.

Although no mass-scale food terrorism case has ever occurred, in the post-9/11 era we live in, it's clear that terrorists are constantly looking for new and unconventional ways to perpetrate attacks. A vulnerable food supply chain could be an effective vehicle for such acts. When he resigned as the secretary of Health and Human Services in 2004, Tommy G. Thompson is often quoted as saying: "For the life of me, I can't understand why the terrorists have not attacked our food supply because it is so easy to do."

Even when they do not cause casualties, food defence issues can badly hurt the finances of food companies at any step of the supply chain. Below are a few examples.

Before food or animals leave the farm.

In 1996 in Wisconsin, pesticide was added to an ingredient used by an animal feed plant. The contaminated feed was then distributed to over 4,000 farms, causing several recalls of dairy products. The convicted person was a competitor of the facility.

http://www3.ntu.edu.sg/rsis/cens/publications/ reports/RSIS_Food%20Defence_170209.pdf (page 12)

After food has left the farm.

In 1978, Palestinian terrorists injected mercury into Israeli oranges. The contamination probably took place at the Dutch port of Rotterdam. The terrorists later declared that they didn't intend to cause any harm to people. https:// www.washingtonpost.com/archive/politics/1978/02/02/ terrorists-poison-israeli-oranges/5650c62a-7ef2-497d-9b20-c47d4376c908/

At the store.

In 2000 in Italy, a terrorist known as "the Italian Unabomber," placed explosives inside several food articles in a large supermarket. No one was ever convicted for those acts.

https://en.wikipedia.org/wiki/Italian_Unabomber

As recently as 2017, a man in Germany contaminated adult and baby food, warning that he would not stop unless he would be paid 11.7m euros. A 53-year old man was later arrested.

https://news.sky.com/story/blackmailer-who-poisoned-baby-food-in-supermarkets-arrested-11061907

As a service to the reader we have created an Excel file containing all the hyperlinks which are mentioned in the book. You can download the Excel file via this link: https://www.foodsafety-experts.com/fsma-book-link/

Alternatively, you can also scan this QR code:

CHAPTER 2

FSMA Overview and Timing

I. HOW FSMA IS MODERNISING THE FOOD SYSTEM

The challenge that FSMA is facing is the scenario of a global food system with no borders and endless connections, where it is often impossible to go back to the exact origins of contaminations and catch frauds. And because complex problems call for complex solutions, the new law had to work on different levels. Let's look at those levels briefly.

It assigns an equal role to prevention.

Prior to FSMA, the food protection system was based on detection and reaction to incidents. It was clear, however, that tests, controls and inspections alone were not enough. Although the law further improves and strengthens that aspect, it also has a new focus on prevention, using two frameworks:

HARPC (Hazard Analysis and Risk-based Controls), which is an expanded version of the traditional HACCP. Overall it is considered more suitable in preventing contaminated food from entering the supply chain;

cGMP (current Good Manufacturing Practices), which received an extensive update before being included in the new law.

We will look at HARCP and cGMP in more detail in chapter 4.

It gives the FDA more power, funding and staffing.

FSMA greatly expands the FDA's range of intervention regarding inspections and administrative detentions. Prior to FSMA, the Agency could only act when it had "credible evidence" of the presence of contaminated food. Now, having "reason to believe" is enough to proceed.

https://www.fda.gov/AnimalVeterinary/Products/AnimalFoodFeeds/ucm347941.htm

FSMA also granted the FDA more funding: in 2011 the Agency's funding gap was $400-450 million. It was reduced to $172 million in 2016. https://www.fda.gov/Food/GuidanceRegulation/FSMA/ucm436160.htm

The whistle-blower program was also strengthened. Employees of food companies are now better protected from retaliation for providing information regarding food safety violations.

It assigns more responsibilities to domestic food operators.

With FSMA, most food operators need to register with the FDA and keep written records for a minimum of two years about all aspects of food manufacturing, processing, packing, receipt, holding or importation. Operators must also keep and implement a written plan for prevention and reaction to food safety incidents.

It requires foreign suppliers to adhere to the same standards of US operators.

FSMA does not only apply to US-based businesses but to any individual, anywhere in the world, who wants to operate in the US food market. Foreign suppliers too, need to be compliant with several provisions of the law and be ready to receive on-site inspections from the FDA. As part of its expanded scope of action, the Agency is required to do at least 600 inspections abroad in the first year and to double that number each year for the next five years. https://www.fda.gov/Food/GuidanceRegulation/FSMA/ucm257978.htm

II. A "WHAT IF" SCENARIO WITH THE PEANUT CORPORATION SALMONELLA OUTBREAK

To give a better idea of how FSMA improved the food system, let's imagine briefly what would have happened with the Peanut Corp Salmonella outbreak if FSMA had been in place at the time.

In the timeline of the case there are two turning points:

- In October 2006, PCA was notified by a customer that one of their products tested positive for Salmonella. The product had also tested positive in the company's internal testing but had been shipped to the customer before the internal lab confirmed the results.

- In January 2009, the FDA started investigating PCA after the Minnesota Department of Health found Salmonella in peanut butter. A few days later, PCA announced the first recall, which was later extended several times.

Under FSMA's rules the customer who found Salmonella in 2006 would have been required to inform the FDA. That would have allowed the Agency to do further inspections and initiate recalls two years earlier. It is fair to say that such a prompt action would have probably saved quite a few lives.

February 15, 2001: A peanut production facility in Blakely, GA operating under the name Casey's Food Products, Inc. changes its name to Peanut Corporation of America. Stewart Parnell takes over as owner and president of the company. Headquarters are established in Lynchburg, Virginia.

June 19, 2003: The Manager of Interim Operations at PCA's Blakely location sends a fax to Daniel Kilgore, the PCA Blakely Operations Manager, instructing him to substitute Chinese Extra-Large Peanuts for Blanched Jumbo Runners when shipping to a customer who had requested the latter, without notifying the customer. These instructions come "per Stewart."

September 2004 – September 2006: During this period, Stewart Parnell and Daniel Kilgore order product to be shipped to customers before receiving results of microbiological testing that reveal the presence of Salmonella in the product on eight separate occasions. They do not inform customers who received the potentially contaminated product in any of these instances.

October 5, 2006: Stewart Parnell is notified by a customer that product received from PCA tested positive for Salmonella. That product is one of those that had tested positive for Salmonella during PCA's internal testing but had been shipped to the customer. Stewart Parnell responds to the customer in an email stating, "<u>I am dumbfounded by what you have found</u>. It is the first time in my over 26 years in the business that I have ever seen any instance of this. We run Certificates of Analysis <u>EVERY DAY</u> with tests for Salmonella and have not found any instances of any, even traces, of a Salmonella problem."

November 16, 2006: Michael Parnell, brother of Stewart Parnell and Vice President of P.P. Sales, the food broker who negotiates sales for PCA, informs Stewart that the company could create a false certificate of analysis if needed.

March 8, 2007: Stewart Parnell sends an email to a customer stating that "We have run countless tests which show absolutely no evidence of Salmonella," referring to a lot of product that he had been informed had tested positive for Salmonella in September 2006.

March 14, 2007: Stewart Parnell sends an email to a customer stating, "Every peanut that we have shipped has only left our facility upon successful negative testing for Salmonella...We can find absolutely no evidence of instances of Salmonella."

March 21, 2007: After being told that Salmonella testing results were not yet available for a lot of product and that shipment would have to be delayed in order to wait for the results, Parnell sends an email that reads: "shit, just ship it. I cannot afford to lose another customer."

April 12, 2007: A PCA official sends an email to the National Sales Manager regarding totes of peanut meal, saying, "They need to air hose the top off though because they are covered in dust and rat crap." The email was forwarded to Stewart Parnell, who replied, "Clean em all up and ship them."

March 2008: Mary Wilkerson is promoted to Quality Assurance Manager at PCA.

March 26, 2008: Daniel Kilgore sends email to Stewart and Michael Parnell regarding testing of peanut paste suggesting that PCA use a smaller sample size "and hope they don't ever catch it."

June 6, 2008: Stewart Parnell sends an email to PCA employees regarding retesting after a presumptive positive Salmonella test on a product. In it he states: "I go through this about once a week...I will hold my breath............again..."

September 2, 2008: Stewart Parnell authorizes Samuel Lightsey, who had taken over from Kilgore as Operations Manager in July of 2008, to ship product that had not tested within acceptable microbiological specifications because the customer didn't require a certificate of analysis.

September 6, 2008: The first victim of what will become a massive Salmonella outbreak linked to PCA products falls ill.

November 10, 2008: The Centre for Disease Control and Prevention (CDC) detects an outbreak of Salmonella Typhimurium, identifying 13 cases in 12 states.

November 24, 2008: CDC identifies a second multistate cluster of Salmonella Typhimurium infections, identifying 27 cases in 14 states.

February 2008 – December 2008: PCA ships 13 lots of peanut products accompanied by false certificates of analysis during this time, later investigations reveal.

February 2008 – January 2009: In later investigations, federal officials discover that peanut products known to be adulterated are introduced into commerce by PCA 20 times during this period.

January 3-4, 2009: CDC pinpoints peanut butter as the likely source of the ongoing Salmonella outbreak.

January 9, 2009: Minnesota Department of Health isolates Salmonella from an opened container of King Nut peanut butter. The U.S. Food and Drug Administration (FDA) launches an investigation of PCA's Blakely, GA facility, where the nut butter was produced.

January 13, 2009: PCA announces a recall of some lots of peanut butter for potential Salmonella contamination.

January 16, 2009: PCA expands its recall to include all peanut butter produced on or after August 8, 2008 and all peanut paste produced on or after September 26, 2008.

January 18, 2009: PCA expands its recall a second time to include all peanut butter and peanut paste manufactured at its Blakely, GA processing plant on or after July 1, 2008.

January 21, 2009: FDA begins investigation of PCA facility in Plainview, TX

January 28, 2009: PCA expands its recall for a third time. All products produced at its Blakely plant since January 1, 2007 are now included.

February 2, 2009: FDA's <u>investigation of PCA's Blakely, GA facility</u> reveals that the plant shipped product before receiving positive test results for Salmonella 12 times between 2007 and 2009.

February 10, 2009: Stewart Parnell appears under subpoena before the House Energy and Commerce Subcommittee during a hearing on the PCA outbreak. He invokes his Fifth Amendment rights and refuses to testify.

February 12, 2009: Texas orders PCA Texas facility to halt production and recall all product manufactured since January 1, 2007. PCA has now recalled over 3,600 products. Over 600 people are now known to have been sickened by Salmonella linked to PCA products.

February 14, 2009: PCA files for Chapter 7 bankruptcy and begins to liquidate its assets.

February 20, 2009: PCA issues a statement to customers telling them to cease distribution of products from PCA plants in Georgia and Texas.

April 2009: The Salmonella outbreak linked to PCA products ends. At least 714 people in 47 states have been sickened. Nine deaths are thought to be attributed to bacteria from PCA peanut products.

March 2010: Stewart Parnell <u>hires</u> Thomas J. Bondurant, Jr. as his defence attorney.

August 26, 2010: A federal judge awards victims of the PCA Salmonella outbreak $12 million in settlement money, to come out of the now-bankrupt PCA's insurance policy.*

> **February 11, 2011**: Family members of victims who died or were sickened in the PCA Salmonella outbreak call for criminal charges to be brought against former PCA officials during a press conference in Washington, D.C.
>
> **October 24, 2012**: Grand Jury subpoenas a former PCA official, a female whose name is kept confidential.
>
> **February 11, 2013**: Daniel Kilgore, Operations Manager at PCA plant in Blakely, GA from June 2002 through May 2008, pleads guilty to one count of conspiracy to commit fraud, one count of conspiracy to introduce adulterated and misbranded food into interstate commerce, eight counts of introducing adulterated food into interstate commerce with the intent to defraud, six counts of introducing misbranded food into interstate commerce with the intent to defraud, eight counts of interstate shipment fraud and five counts of wire fraud. See court documents here.
>
> **February 21, 2013**: The Justice Department files a 76-count indictment of former PCA officials, including Stewart Parnell, Michael Parnell, Samuel Lightsey and Mary Wilkerson.

III. HOW FSMA IS ORGANISED

FSMA is a complex law with many parts. To make navigation easier, here is an overview of how it is organised from top to bottom.

The titles of the Law

The full text of the original Act of Law can be found here. However, reading it is not for the layman. It is written as a continuous list of references and amendments to the existing Federal Food, Drug, and Cosmetic Act of 1938. However, it is clearly divided into four Titles, which cover the areas of intervention we mentioned at the beginning of this chapter:

- improving capacity to prevent food safety problems (Title I);
- improving capacity to detect and respond to food safety problems (Title II);
- improving the safety of imported food (Title III);
- miscellaneous provisions about FDA funding, employee protection and international cooperation (Title IV).

The seven foundational rules

Following a period of public comments, the FDA translated the law into several implementable rules for its application in the real world. All rules are part of Title 21 of the Code of Federal Regulations, dedicated to Food and Drugs. There are seven foundational rules in FSMA.

Current cGMP and HARPC for Human Food.

It sets the rules to implement a prevention-oriented system based on HARPC and cGMP. It was published on 17 Sept 2015 and came into effect on 16 Nov 2015.

https://www.ecfr.gov/cgi-bin/text-idx?SID=a08332439ea5c 8d24f270c2f6c95fc84&mc=true&node=pt21.2.117&rgn=div5

Current cGMP and HARPC for Animal Food.

It is also based on HARPC and cGMP and regulates food for animal consumption. It was published on 17 Sept 2015 and came into effect on 16 Nov 2015.

https://www.ecfr.gov/cgi-bin/text-idx?SID=a08332439ea5c8d24f270c2f6c95fc84&mc=true&node=pt21.6.507&rgn=div5

Mitigation Strategies to Protect Food Against Intentional Adulteration.

The rule is for the prevention of wide-spread acts of intentional adulteration and mainly applies to large companies. It was published on 27 May 2016 and came into effect on 26 July 2016.

https://www.ecfr.gov/cgi-bin/text-idx?SID=a08332439ea5c8d24f270c2f6c95fc84&mc=true&node=pt21.2.121&rgn=div5

Foreign Supplier Verification Program for Food Importers (FSVP).

The rule is directed to all operators importing food to the US as well as to foreign suppliers. It was published on 27 Nov 2015 and came into effect on 26 Jan 2016.

https://www.ecfr.gov/cgi-bin/text-idx?SID=a08332439ea5c8d24f270c2f6c95fc84&mc=true&node=sp21.1.1.l&rgn=div6

Sanitary Transportation of Human and Animal Food.

It sets the rules and practices to prevent food safety issues during transportation of food. It was published on 6 Apr 2016 and came into effect on 6 June 2016.

https://www.ecfr.gov/cgi-bin/text-idx?SID=a08332439ea5c8d24f270c2f6c95fc84&mc=true&node=sp21.1.1.o&rgn=div6

Accreditation of Third-Party Certification Bodies to Conduct Food Safety Audits and to Issue Certifications.

It is a subpart of the rule on General Enforcement Regulations which establishes a voluntary program for the accreditation of third-party auditors. It was published on 27 November 2015 and came into effect on 26 January 2016.

https://www.ecfr.gov/cgi-bin/text-idx?SID=a08332439ea 5c8d24f270c2f6c95fc84&mc=true&node=pt21.1.1&rgn=di v5#sp21.1.1.m

Standards for the Growing, Harvesting, Packing, and Holding of Produce for Human Consumption.

The rule sets minimum standards for growing and treating fruits and vegetables for human consumption. It was published on 27 Nov 2015 and came into effect on 26 Jan 2016.

https://www.ecfr.gov/cgi-bin/text-idx?SID=a08332439ea 5c8d24f270c2f6c95fc84&mc=true&node=pt21.2.112&rgn =div5

The *Voluntary Qualified Importer Program (VQIP)* is another important part in FSMA. It is a voluntary fee-based program that helps importers speed-up the review and entry process of human and animal food. It started accepting applications on 31 January 2018.

https://www.fda.gov/Food/GuidanceRegulation/ ImportsExports/Importing/ucm490823.htm

We'll examine each of these parts in detail in the following chapters. The only exception will be the rule on Third-party

Certification: this book is targeted at producers and growers in the food industry, so it would be out of scope.

Guidelines

The FDA also published industry guidelines, which describe the rules in a more accessible language. They come with a disclaimer that they should be considered as a series of recommendations rather than legally binding provisions.

IV. WHO IS SUBJECT TO THE LAW?

FSMA is a complex law, so there is no short answer to that question. Complex, however, does not mean unclear. Indeed, FSMA defines in detail who needs to comply with each rule, although it still leaves some room for a case-by-case approach.

The best way to introduce the aspect of applicability is to look at the definitions of the main operators affected by the law: farms, facilities, transporters, importers and suppliers.

Farms

The most basic difference between farms and facilities is that farms grow and harvest food, while facilities are dedicated to processing and manufacturing it. There are, however, a few nuances to consider.

Farms are divided into **primary** and **secondary**. *Primary farms* are operations under **one management** and **one location** (although not necessarily contiguous), and are dedicated to primary farming activities such as:

- growing crops;
- harvesting crops;
- raising animals, including seafood;
- any combination of the above.

Additionally, primary farms may also include processing activities such as:

- packing of holding of raw agricultural commodities (RACs), whether they were grown in the farm or not;
- manufacturing/processing of food and packing or holding of processed food, if it is consumed on that farm or another farm under the same management;
- manufacturing/processing of food and packing or holding of processed food that is *not* consumed on the farm, <u>provided that the processing activities are limited to</u>:
  - o Drying/dehydrating, packaging and labelling RACs to create a distinct commodity, without additional manufacturing/processing
  - o Ripening RACs (also artificially with ethylene gas) without additional manufacturing/processing.

Practical examples

Below are a few examples of primary farms that can perform additional activities without triggering the facility definition.

- A primary farm aggregates RACs from both its own farming activity and other farms, for distribution through a Community Supported Agriculture (CSA) model, e.g. a U-pick set-up or a farm selling at farmer's markets.

- A farmer keeps part of the RACs grown at the farm for the consumption of his family or animals.
- A farm that has a coffee shop selling coffee and cakes will be allowed to do any type of food processing activity (baking, grinding, squeezing etc.), both on ingredients grown and harvested at the farm itself (apples for cakes for example), or from other suppliers (flour, eggs, coffee, etc.) and still be considered a farm. Any processed food however, *cannot leave the farm unconsumed.*
- A farm grows and dehydrates grapes to make raisins and sells them to a distributor.
- A farm grows kiwis and stores them for ripening before selling them.

By contrast, a farm that sells dehydrated sliced mushrooms would fall outside the farm definition, because slicing is not part of the short list of allowed processing activities.

A secondary farm is an operation with the following characteristics:

- It is not located on a primary production farm (meaning it is separated from the primary farm by more than a patch of land or a road);
- It is not dedicated to growing crops, but performs other farming activities such as harvesting, packing, and/or holding of RACs;
- the majority of its interests are owned by one or more primary farms jointly;
- the primary farm (or farms) owning the operation must provide the majority of the RACs that are harvested, packed or held by the operation.

Similarly to primary farms, secondary farms may also manufacture/process food, and hold and pack processed food, with the same limitations of primary farms.

Practical example

Different independent farms form a cooperative to share harvesting costs. This cooperative is not located on any of the primary farms that own it. As an additional source of revenue, it also harvests RACs for other farms, but the harvested quantity from this additional activity is less than 50% of total harvested RACs.

Facilities and farm mixed-type facilities

Simply put, food facilities are operations that manufacture and process food. The FDA's official definition for these two activities is:

Making food from one or more ingredients, or synthesizing, preparing, treating, modifying or manipulating food, including food crops or ingredients.

The FDA also gives a list of examples of specific manufacturing and processing activities, such as freezing, grinding, pasteurizing, etc.

As we have seen, in FSMA some processing activities like drying/dehydrating, ripening, labelling, packing, belong to the 'farm' definition. The line that separates farms from facilities can therefore be subtle.

Consider the example of a farm that grows and harvests peanuts. The farm can leave them to dry (a process known as 'curing') and still be considered a farm. Removing them from the shells however, would be a processing activity. Similarly, a farm can harvest plums and dehydrate them, but removing the seeds would be a processing activity.

Farms are of course free to engage in any type of processing activities. In that case however, they would be considered *farm mixed-type facilities*, and their processing activities would be subject to the same rules of other facilities.

Transporters

FSMA defines **food transportation** as all transportation activities within the US, either by road or rail, "that may affect the sanitary condition of food." There are four types of individuals involved in food transportation:

- the **shipper**, who arranges the transportation, whether it is the manufacturer or a freight broker;
- the **loader**, who loads the food onto a vehicle;
- the **carrier,** who physically moves the food;
- the **receiver,** who receives the food, whether at its final destination or anywhere in between.

There are, however, a few important specifications and exceptions to keep in mind:

- the definition of shipper also includes those who ship food by ship or air, as long as the food is then transferred by motor or rail to be consumed or distributed within the US;
- if the food is being transferred *through* the US by motor or rail to a destination abroad and the container remains intact, then the food is not subject to FSMA;

- the definition of carrier excludes those who deliver food to final consumers ("parcel delivery service").

The list of exceptions does not end here. We will look at them more in detail in chapter 10.

Importers

The importer is the US owner of, or the person who, receives an article of food offered for import into the US. "Offered for import" means that the importer may:

- own the food;
- have purchased it, or
- have agreed in writing to purchase it.

For this definition, it is crucial that the importer is *based in the US*. In case the owner or the consignee is foreign (a less frequent case), the law will consider their US agent or representative as importers, but that relationship needs to be confirmed by a signed statement of consent.

There are exceptions to this definition as well. We will look at them in detail in chapter 6.

Foreign suppliers

A foreign food supplier is an establishment that comes last in the supply chain before the food is exported to the US. The definition excludes those entities that only perform activities that do not change the state of the exported food (e.g. labelling).

The FDA conducts regular inspections on foreign food facilities, based on three factors: the food safety risk associated with the type of food, the manufacturing process, and the compliance history of the facility.

Exemptions

For each of the FSMA rules there are specific exemptions. All of the exemptions will be discussed in the relevant, subsequent chapters where we will discuss the requirements of each FSMA rule in more detail.

V. REGISTERING WITH THE FDA

Any facility, including those outside the US, which intends to process, pack or hold food for the US market must register with the FDA. This mandatory step was introduced in the 2002 Bioterrorism Act, in the aftermath of the 9/11 attacks.

Registration must be renewed biannually, every even year between the 1st of October and the end of December. Missing these dates might mean losing the registration and being fined by the FDA.

Facilities can register directly with the FDA for free using this link https://www.fda.gov/Food/GuidanceRegulation/FoodFacilityRegistration/default.htm, or

through a private company called, RegistrarCorp, for a fee of $100: https://www.registrarcorp.com/fda-food/

Who is exempt from registration

The following food operators are exempt from registering with the FDA:

- Farms, both primary and secondary. Farm mixed-type facilities, however, are required to register
- Restaurants
- Retail food establishments (see full definition in CFR §1.227)
- Facilities that only handle meat, poultry, or egg products, which are overseen by the USDA
- Non-profit establishments that prepare or serve food directly to people (like food banks or soup kitchens)
- Fishing vessels, including those that perform certain minimal processing activities in addition to harvesting and transporting fish

VI. BUSINESS SIZES ACCORDING TO FSMA

Other than the type of activities, FSMA also uses business size to categorise food operations and assign different types of provisions. There are up to three size categories: very small, small and large, and the exact criteria vary depending on the type of operator.

Types of farms by size

With farms, FSMA considers the rolling annual average value (adjusted for inflation) of produce sold in the previous three-year period. Based on that value, a farm is:

- very small if it is up to $250,000;
- small if it is between $250,001 and $500,000;
- large, if it is above $500,000.

Types of facilities by size

For food facilities, FSMA's criteria are a mix of turnover value and number of employees. They can be:

- very small businesses, if the rolling annual average value (adjusted for inflation) of human food in the previous three-year period is less than $1 million for human food and $2.5 for animal food. The calculation includes the market value of both sold food and food held without sale;
- small businesses, if they have fewer than 500 full-time equivalent employees;
- large businesses, if they have more than 500 full-time equivalent employees.

Types of importers by size

For importers, FSMA only distinguishes between very small businesses and everybody else. In this case, the same criteria for very small facilities apply, both for human and animal food.

VII. COMPLIANCE TIMELINE BY BUSINESS SIZE

One of the most immediate implications of business size are compliance dates.

As expected, such a complex law like FSMA was implemented in several steps, allowing to all affected operations a grace period to comply with its provisions. The full overview can be found on the FDA website: https://www.fda.gov/downloads/Food/GuidanceRegulation/FSMA/UCM568798.pdf

Let's look at compliance dates in details by business size.

VERY SMALL BUSINESSES

2015	2016	2017	2018	2019	2020	2021
SEP 17, 2015 (PCHF) Preventive Controls Human Food Final Rule Published	JAN 01, 2016 (PCHF) Very Small Businesses retain records to support Qualified Facility status	JAN 01, 2017 (PCAF) Very Small Businesses retain records to support Qualified Facility Status	MAR 19, 2018 (FSVP)1,6 Importer of human food whose Small Business Foreign Supplier required to comply with PCHF	MAR 18, 2019 (FSVP)1,6 Importer of animal food whose Small Business Foreign Supplier is subject to the PC requirements in PCAF, but not the CGMP requirements	MAR 17, 2020 (FSVP)1,6 Importer of animal food whose Foreign Supplier is a Qualified Facility (including Very Small Businesses) subject to PCAF PC, but not CGMP requirements	JUL 26, 2021 (IA) Very Small Business
SEP 17, 2015 (PCAF) Preventive Controls Animal Food Final Rule Published	JAN 26 2016 (FSVP) FSVP Effective Date	MAY 30, 2017 (FSVP)1,6 Importer not subject to PC or produce rules	MAR 19, 2018 (FSVP)1,6 Importer of animal food whose Large Business Foreign Supplier is subject to the PC requirements in PCAF, but not the CGMP requirements	MAR 18, 2019 (FSVP)1,6 Importer of human food Grade "A" milk and milk products whose foreign supplier is subject to PMO requirements	JUL 27, 2020 (FSVP)1,6 Importer whose Very Small Business Foreign Supplier subject to Produce Safety Rule and eligible for a Qualified Exemption	
NOV 16, 2015 (PCHF) Preventive Controls Human Food Effective Date	MAY 27, 2016 (IA) Intentional Adulteration Final Rule Published	MAY 30, 2017 (FSVP)1,6 Importer of human food whose Large Foreign Supplier required to comply with PCHF	MAR 19, 2018 (FSVP)1,6 Importer of animal food whose Small Business Foreign Supplier is subject to PCAF CGMP requirements	MAR 18, 2019 (FSVP)1,6 Importer of human food whose Foreign Supplier is a Qualified Facility (including Very Small Businesses)	JUL 27, 2020 (FSVP)1,6 Importer whose Very Small Business Foreign Supplier is subject to the produce safety rule	
NOV 16, 2015 (PCAF) Preventive Controls Animal Food Effective Date	JUL 26, 2016 (IA) Intentional Adulteration Effective Date	MAY 30, 2017 (FSVP)1,6 Importer of animal food whose Large Foreign Supplier is subject to PCAF CGMP requirements	JUL 26, 2018 (FSVP)1,6 Importer whose Small Business Foreign Supplier required to comply with sprout requirements of Produce Safety Rule	MAR 18, 2019 (FSVP)1,6 Importer of animal food whose Foreign Supplier is a Qualified Facility (including Very Small Businesses) subject to PCAF CGMP requirements		
NOV 27, 2015 (FSVP) Foreign Supplier Verification Program Final Rule Published		JUL 26, 2017 (FSVP)1,6 Importer whose Large Foreign Supplier required to comply with sprout requirements of Produce Safety Rule	JUL 26, 2018 (FSVP)1,6 Importer whose Small Business Foreign Supplier is a farm producing sprouts and eligible for a Qualified Exemption under the Produce Safety Rule	JUL 29, 2019 (FSVP-1,6 Importer whose Very Small Business Foreign Supplier is a farm producing sprouts and eligible for a Qualified Exemption under the Produce Safety Rule		
			JUL 26, 2018 (FSVP)1,6 Importer whose Large Foreign Supplier Required to comply with Produce Safety Rule	JUL 29, 2019 (FSVF)1,6 Importer whose Small Business Foreign Supplier required to comply with Produce Safety Rule		
			SEP 17, 2018 (PCHF)2,3,4 Qualified Facilities (including Very Small Businesses) compliance	JUL 29, 2019 (FSVP)1,6 Importer whose Small Business Foreign Supplier subject to Produce Safety Rule and eligible for a Qualified Exemption		
			SEP 17, 2018 (PCHF) Grade "A" milk and milk products subject to the Pasteurized Milk Ordinance (PMO)	JUL 29, 2019 (FSVP)1,6 Importer whose Very Small Business Foreign Supplier required to comply with Sprout Requirements of Produce Safety Rule		
			SEP 17, 2018 (PCAF)2,3 Qualified facilities (including Very Small Businesses) CGMP compliance	SEP 17, 2019 (PCAF)2,3,5 Qualified Facilities (including Very Small Businesses) PC Compliance		

SMALL BUSINESSES

2015	2016	2017	2018	2019	2020
SEP 17, 2015 (PCHF) Preventive Controls Human Food Final Rule Published	JAN 26, 2016 (FSVP) FSVP Effective Date	MAY 30, 2017 (FSVP)1,6 Importer not subject to PC or produce rules	MAR 19, 2018 (FSVP)1,6 Importer of human food whose Small Business Foreign Supplier required to comply with PCHF	MAR 18, 2019 (FSVP)1,6 Importer of animal food whose Small Business Foreign Supplier is subject to the PC requirements in PCAF, but not the CGMP requirements	MAR 17, 2020 (FSVP)1,6 Importer of animal food whose Foreign Supplier is a Qualified Facility (including Very Small Businesses) subject to PCAF PC, but not CGMP requirements
SEP 17, 2015 (PCAF) Preventive Controls Animal Food Final Rule Published	APR 06, 2016 (ST) Sanitary Transportation of Human and Animal Food Final Rule Published	MAY 30, 2017 (FSVP)1,6 Importer of human food whose Large Foreign Supplier required to comply with PCHF	MAR 19, 2018 (FSVP)1,6 Importer of animal food whose Large Business Foreign Supplier is subject to the PC requirements in PCAF, but not the CGMP requirements	MAR 18, 2019 (FSVP)1,6 Importer of human food Grade "A" milk and milk products whose foreign supplier is subject to PMO requirements	JUL 27, 2020 (IA) Small Business
NOV 16, 2015 (PCHF) Preventive Controls Human Food Effective Date	MAY 27, 2016 (IA) Intentional Adulteration Final Rule Published	MAY 30, 2017 (FSVP)1,6 Importer of animal food whose Large Foreign Supplier is subject to PCAF CGMP requirements	MAR 19, 2018 (FSVP)1,6 Importer of animal food whose Small Business Foreign Supplier is subject to PCAF CGMP requirements	MAR 18, 2019 (FSVP)1,6 Importer of human food whose Foreign Supplier is a Qualified Facility (including Very Small Businesses)	JUL 27, 2020 (FSVP)1,6 Importer whose Very Small Business Foreign Supplier subject to Produce Safety Rule and eligible for a Qualified Exemption
NOV 16, 2015 (PCAF) Preventive Controls Animal Food Effective Date	JUN 06, 2016 (ST) Sanitary Transportation Effective Date	JUL 26, 2017 (FSVP)1,6 Importer whose Large Foreign Supplier required to comply with sprout requirements of Produce Safety Rule	APR 06, 2018 (ST) Small Business	MAR 18, 2019 (FSVP)1,6 Importer of animal food whose Foreign Supplier is a Qualified Facility (including Very Small Businesses) subject to PCAF CGMP requirements	JUL 27, 2020 (FSVP)1,6 Importer whose Very Small Business Foreign Supplier is subject to the produce safety rule
NOV 27, 2015 (FSVP) Foreign Supplier Verification Program Final Rule Published	JUL 26, 2016 (IA) Intentional Adulteration Effective Date	SEP 18, 2017 (PCHF)1,2,3,4 Small Business compliance	JUL 26, 2018 (FSVP)1,6 Importer whose Small Business Foreign Supplier required to comply with sprout requirements of Produce Safety Rule		
		SEP 18, 2017 (PCAF)2,3 Small Business CGMP compliance	JUL 26, 2018 (FSVP)1,6 Importer whose Small Business Foreign Supplier is a farm producing sprouts and eligible for a Qualified Exemption under the Produce Safety Rule		
			JUL 26, 2018 (FSVP)1,6 Importer whose Large Foreign Supplier Required to comply with Produce Safety Rule		

LARGE BUSINESSES

2015	2016	2017	2018	2019	2020
SEP 17, 2015 (PCHF) Preventive Controls Human Food Final Rule Published	JAN 26, 2016 (FSVP) FSVP Effective Date	APR 06, 2017 (ST) Large Business	MAR 19, 2018 (FSVP)1,6 Importer of human food whose Small Business Foreign Supplier required to comply with PCHF	MAR 18, 2019 (FSVP)1,6 Importer of human food whose Small Business Foreign Supplier is subject to the PC requirements in PCAF, but not the CGMP requirements	MAR 17, 2020 (FSVP)1,6 Importer of animal food whose Foreign Supplier is a Qualified Facility (including Very Small Businesses) subject to PCAF PC, but not CGMP requirements
SEP 17, 2015 (PCAF) Preventive Controls Animal Food Final Rule Published	APR 06, 2016 (ST) Sanitary Transportation of Human and Animal Food Final Rule Published	MAY 30, 2017 (FSVP)1,6 Importer of human food whose Large Foreign Supplier required to comply with PCHF	MAR 19, 2018 (FSVP)1,6 Importer of animal food whose Large Business Foreign Supplier is subject to the PC requirements in PCAF, but not the CGMP requirements	MAR 18, 2019 (FSVP)1,6 Importer of human food Grade "A" milk and milk products whose foreign supplier is subject to PMO requirements	JUL 27, 2020 (FSVP)1,6 Importer whose Very Small Business Foreign Supplier subject to Produce Safety Rule and eligible for a Qualified Exemption
NOV 16, 2015 (PCHF) Preventive Controls Human Food Effective Date	MAY 27, 2016 (IA) Intentional Adulteration Final Rule Published	MAY 30, 2017 (FSVP)1,6 Importer of animal food whose Large Foreign Supplier is subject to PCAF CGMP requirements	MAR 19, 2018 (FSVP)1,6 Importer of animal food whose Small Business Foreign Supplier is subject to PCAF CGMP requirements	MAR 18, 2019 (FSVP)1,6 Importer of human food whose Foreign Supplier is a Qualified Facility (including Very Small Businesses)	JUL 27, 2020 (FSVP)1,6 Importer whose Very Small Business Foreign Supplier is subject to the produce safety rule
NOV 16, 2015 (PCAF) Preventive Controls Animal Food Effective Date	JUN 06, 2016 (ST) Sanitary Transportation Effective Date	JUL 26, 2017 (FSVP)1,6 Importer whose Large Foreign Supplier required to comply with sprout requirements of Produce Safety Rule	JUL 26, 2018 (FSVP)1,6 Importer whose Small Business Foreign Supplier required to comply with sprout requirements of Produce Safety Rule	MAR 18, 2019 (FSVP)1,6 Importer of animal food whose Foreign Supplier is a Qualified Facility (including Very Small Businesses)	
NOV 27, 2015 (FSVP) Foreign Supplier Verification Program Final Rule Published	JUL 25, 2016 (IA) Intentional Adulteration Effective Date	SEP 18, 2017 (PCAF)1,2,3,5 Large Business PC compliance	JUL 26, 2018 (FSVP)1,6 Importer whose Small Business Foreign Supplier is a farm producing sprouts and eligible for a Qualified Exemption under the Produce Safety Rule	JUL 26, 2019 (IA) Large Business	
	SEP 19, 2016 (PCHF)1,2,3,4 Large Business		JUL 26, 2018 (FSVP)1,6 Importer whose Large Foreign Supplier Required to comply with Produce Safety Rule	JUL 29, 2019 (FSVP)1,6 Importer whose Small Business Foreign Supplier is a farm producing sprouts and eligible for a Qualified Exemption under the Produce Safety Rule	
	SEP 19, 2016 (PCAF)2,3 Large Business CGMP compliance		SEP 17, 2018 (PCHF) Grade "A" milk and milk products subject to the Pasteurized Milk Ordinance (PMO)	JUL 29, 2019 (FSVP)1,6 Importer whose Small Business Foreign Supplier required to comply with Produce Safety Rule	
				JUL 29, 2019 (FSVP)1,6 Importer whose Small Business Foreign Supplier subject to Produce Safety Rule and eligible for a Qualified Exemption	
				JUL 29, 2019 (FSVP)1,6 Importer whose Very Small Business Foreign Supplier required to comply with Sprout Requirements of Produce Safety Rule	

VIII. COMPARING FSMA WITH GFSI

The Preventive Controls rule includes many requirements. However, if an organisation is already certified by one GFSI's food safety management schemes, the to-do list is likely to be shorter than expected. Here below is an overview of the major differences between FSMA requirements and each of the four major GFSI scheme's standards.

FSSC 22000

The Archeson Group created a comparison between the FSMA requirements and FSSC 22000. The summary table of the report is shown below. The full report can be downloaded via this link: http://www.fssc22000.com/documents/pdf/2016-tag-analysis-human-food-final-april-2016.pdf

Key areas	FDA Preventive Controls Food Safety Plan	FDA GMPs (117 Subpart B)	FSSC 22000 Scheme Equivalence
1. Overarching Policy Statement	No	No	Yes (Exceeds)
2. Written Plan	Yes	No	Yes (Comparable)
3. Experienced Individual in Charge	Yes	No	Yes (Comparable in qualifications; Exceeds in responsibility)
4. Trained Staff	Yes	Yes	Yes (Comparable)
5. Prerequisite Programs	No	Yes	Yes (Exceeds)
6. Raw Material/ Incoming Product Safety Assurance	No	No	Yes (Exceeds)
7. Supplier Verification	Yes	No	Yes (Comparable)
8. Allergen Management	Yes	Yes	Yes (Comparable)
9. Validation of Controls	Yes	No	Yes (Comparable)
10. Finished Product Testing	No	No	Yes (Exceeds)
11. Sanitation Control	Yes	Yes	Yes (Exceeds)
12. Corrective Actions	Yes	No	Yes (Comparable)
13. Traceability	No[1]	No	Yes (Comparable)
14. Recall	Yes	No	Yes (Comparable)
15. Record Retention	Yes	No	Yes (Different)
16. Food Defense	No[2]	No	Yes (Exceeds)
17. Internal Audit & Management Review	No[3]	No	Yes (Exceeds)

[1] FDA has already established traceability requirements under regulation stemming from the 2002 Bioterrorism Act, and traceability is a component of sec 204 FMSA which is separate from Preventive Controls
[2] Although FSMA addresses food defense in sec 103, FDA issued a separate rule on Intentional Adulteration while the final rule is expected by May 2016
[3] Some of the record review requirements accomplish similar objectives to the internal audit

Record Retention. The main differences are in the area of record retention. The FSSC 22000 standard requires that records demonstrating compliance with procedures and process control be retained for as long as necessary to meet customers' or legal requirements. FSMA, by contrast has a general two-year retention requirement (except for documentation related to qualified facilities exemption). The solution in this case is to adopt the longer of the two options: legal or customer-based retention or the minimum of 2 years retention as dictated by FSMA.

SQF

The Archeson Group provided a good comparison between SQF and FSMA requirements. The summary table is shown below, and the detailed report can be downloaded via this link: https://www.sqfi.com/wp-content/uploads/Produce-safety-rule-comparison-to-SQF.pdf

	SQF – Level 2	FDA Preventive Controls Food Safety Plan	FDA GMPs (117 subpart B)
Overarching policy statement	Yes	No	No
Written Plan	Yes	Yes	No
Experienced individual in charge	Yes	Yes	No
Trained Staff	Yes	Yes*	Yes
Prerequisite programs	Yes	No	Yes
Raw material/ incoming product safety assurance	Yes	No	No
Supplier Verification	Yes	Yes, in specific cases**	No
Allergen Management	Yes	Yes	Yes
Validation of Controls	Yes	Yes	No
Finished product testing	No	Yes, in specific cases**	No
Sanitation Control	Yes	Yes	Yes
Environmental monitoring	Yes	Yes, in specific cases**	No
Corrective Actions	Yes	Yes	No
Traceability	Yes	No[1]	No
Recall	Yes	Yes	No
Record retention	Yes	Yes	No
Food defense	Yes	No[2]	No
Internal Audit	Yes	No[3]	No

[1] FDA has already established traceability requirements under regulation stemming from the 2002 Bioterrorism Act, and traceability is a component of sec 204 FMSA which is separate from the Final Preventive Controls Rule
[2] FSMA addresses food defense in Sec 103. FDA has released a proposed rule pertaining to intentional contamination that will stand separately and finalize in 2016.
[3] Some of the record review requirements accomplish similar objectives to the internal audit

There are two big differences around validation of controls and corrective actions.

Validation of Controls. Validation and effectiveness of preventive controls in FSMA go beyond SQF requirements in specifying that records must be on site for 6 months and retained for two years. Also, the food safety plan needs to be re-analysed every 3 years and in other specified circumstances (as will be discussed in chapter 4 in more detail). Prerequisite programs are not required to be validated by FSMA unless these are elevated to a preventative control requiring validation.

Corrective actions. Both SQF and FSMA require a documented process to manage corrective actions. FSMA, however includes more details as it specifically requires an evaluation of the food in question and assurance that potentially contaminated food has not entered commerce. An easy solution to this is to always block the available stock in case of a corrective action and determine whether there are more affected products that have already been shipped to (other) customers.

BRC

As with the other GFSI certification schemes, companies that are already compliant with BRC issue 7 will have to make adaptations in the identification of preventative controls and assigning a Preventive Controls Qualified Individual.

Identification of "Preventive Controls." The BRC certification is based on the traditional HACCP approach, while the PC rule is based on HARPC. The main difference will be with plant environmental controls, which are part of HARPC, but are considered a prerequisite in HACCP. To be HARPC-compliant, BRC sites will have to reassess their prerequisites (e.g. Cleaning and Sanitation, Allergen Control, etc.) under FSMA's guidelines, and represent them as "Preventive Controls."

Identification of a Qualified Individual (PCQI). FSMA requires each site to identify a Qualified Individual (ideally the Quality Assurance Manager) who is fully trained in the application of the HARPC process.

BRC included all details of the necessary changes in a nice booklet that can be downloaded via this link:

https://www.brcglobalstandards.com/media/48150/ brctag-guidance-document.pdf It is also possible to request an additional module which will be formally audited and recorded in BRC's audit report. This can be an effective way to prove compliance with FSMA.

IFS

IFS asked Neumann Risk Services to make a comparison between FSMA and the IFS requirements. The full report can be downloaded via this link: www.exaris.fr/loadDoc. php?id=6753

The abstract is shown in the table below:

2.2.3.5 Hazard analysis requirements	The hazard analysis process required by IFS and FDA are comparable, but the Preventative Control Rules include significantly more detail as to how the analysis process is to be undertaken. For example, FDA specifically requires an evaluation of environmental pathogens whenever a ready-to-eat food is exposed to the environment prior to packaging and the packaging food does not receive a treatment that would minimize the pathogen.
5.3 Process Validation and Control	The PC Rule contains detailed guidelines for monitoring and validation of preventative controls that are more prescriptive than the process validation and control requirements in the IFS Standards.
5.4 Calibration	The PC rule requires calibration of monitoring instruments and sets forth specific requirements on what records must be kept, and how frequently those records relating to calibration must be reviewed. The IFS Rule requires that calibration records be maintained. However, it does not specifically require that these records be reviewed or specify how frequently to review records relating to calibration. The PC rule does not specifically require calibration against a national or international reference standard.
5.11 Corrective Actions	FDA's requirements regarding corrective actions and corrections are more prescriptive and detailed. For example, FDA requires specific written corrective action procedures to be developed addressing the presence of pathogens in ready-to-eat products. FDA also describes in detail the steps that must be included within the corrective action procedures.

The main differences are in relation to the hazards analysis requirements, process validation and control, calibration and corrective actions.

Hazard analysis. FSMA's hazard analysis process is more detailed, for example in the evaluation of environmental pathogens whenever a ready-to-eat food is exposed to the environment prior to packaging and the packaged food does not get an additional treatment.

Process Validation and Control. The guidelines of the PC Rule are more prescriptive.

Calibration. The PC rule has detailed requirements on the calibration of monitoring instruments and review and retention of records.

Corrective Actions. FDA's requirements are more prescriptive and detailed, for example regarding the presence of pathogens in ready-to-eat products.

As a service to the reader we have created an Excel file containing all the hyperlinks which are mentioned in the book. You can download the Excel file via this link: https://www.foodsafety-experts.com/fsma-book-link/

Alternatively, you can also scan this QR code:

CHAPTER 3

Creating Your Implementation Plan

In the following even numbered chapters of this book, each of the FSMA rules will be explained in detail. The uneven numbered chapters (5,7,9,11 and 13) have been inserted to provide a personalised implementation plan for your organisation in order to become FSMA compliant. Each of the uneven chapters contains a table with the following columns:

- Company Size – t specifies the required actions based on the size of your organization (big, small or very small). Most tables start with the items which are relevant for all company sizes.
- Item description – it gives a brief description of the aspect of the FSMA rule which needs to be implemented or verified.

- Relevant – here you can document whether this item is relevant for your organization.
- Action – here you can document the action which you are (or someone else is) going to take in your organization.
- Remarks – it contains additional remarks for further clarification.
- Responsible – here you can document the responsible person for each action.
- Due Date – here you can document the due date for each action.
- Status – here you can provide an update on each action item as it is being progressed over time.

Of course, you will only need to use the relevant chapters for your organisation, e.g. Chapters 4 and 5 if you produce human food or animal food, or Chapters 12 and 13 for agricultural commodities. To aid implementation even more, we have created an Excel file containing all of the tables of the uneven chapters. You can download it via this link: https://www.foodsafety-experts.com/fsma-book-excel/. Alternatively you can scan this QR-code:

At the end of the even chapters, we included a link to our website where, after registration, you can find all the links mentioned in the chapter. As over time some of them might become obsolete, we have copied all of the information to our servers and you can access this information via our website. Upon registration you will be asked for a specific word from this book, so have your book at hand (or on screen if you have the Kindle version) for your registration.

For those of you who want even more information, such as templates for procedures and records, additional material in relation to exporting to the USA, and enforcement by the FDA, we kindly refer you to our on-line FSMA Masterclass. For more information, you can go to this link: https://foodsafety-university.thinkific.com/courses/fsma-masterclass. Alternatively, you can scan this QR-code:

CHAPTER 4

Preventive Controls for Human and Animal Food

I. HOW THE PC RULE IS STRUCTURED

F SMA has two separate rules for preventive controls: one for human food (CFR §117) and one for animal food (CFR §507), which are, for the most part, similar. For the sake of simplicity, in this chapter we will describe the rule on Preventive Controls for Human Food, with the assumption that the same provisions apply to animal food. Significant differences will be added in the separate boxes below.

The rule on Preventive Controls for Human Food is divided into seven subparts, marked with letters from A to G.

A. General Provisions. It lays down the preliminary concepts and definitions of the rule, specifies its applicability, and what records need to be maintained.

This section in the Preventive Controls for Animal Food rule (PCAF) contains a reference to the Preventive Controls for Human Food rule (PCHF) for mixed type facilities.

In PCAF there is no reference to allergen cross-contamination.

In terms of qualification of individuals, the process is similar but PCHF focuses on human food where PCAF focuses on animal food for training.

PCAF §507.7 - *Requirements that apply to a qualified facility* - matches with PCHF §117.201 on *Modified requirements that apply to a qualified facility*, which is in a different section.

In PCAF the scope of Supply Chain Control and HARPC is reduced. While in PCHF they include all unexposed human food, in PCAF they only apply when the unexposed animal food does not require temperature control to reduce the risk of microbiological hazards.

PCAF §507.12 - *Applicability of this part to the holding and distribution of human food by-products for use as animal food* - states that if a human food plant or farm also produces animal feed by-products without further processing, the facility is exempt from the PCAF rule.

PCHF §117.9 - *Records required for this subpart* - is included in PCAF §507.4 - *Qualifications of individuals who manufacture, process, pack, or hold animal food.*

B. Current Good Manufacturing Practice. These are the foundational practices to ensure safe processing of food in the facility. This subpart includes a detailed description of every aspect of cGMP, from staff procedures to warehousing and distribution.

In PCAF there are no requirements related to the following aspects of food contact surfaces: allergen cross-contamination, smooth bonding of connecting surfaces and mandatory visual display of temperature measurement in fridges and freezers.

PCAF has fewer requirements related to the heating steps designed to reduce the impact of microbiological contaminants.

PCAF includes no requirements to prevent cross-contamination with physical, chemical, microbiological, radiological and allergen hazards in warehousing.

PCHF §117.95 - Holding and distribution of human food by-products for use as animal food – is comprised in the following two sections of PCAF:

- *§507.27 - Holding and distribution.*

- *§507.28 - Holding and distribution of human food by-products for use as animal food.*

C. Hazard Analysis and Risk-Based Preventive Controls. The purpose of HARPC is to minimise or eliminate the risk of food safety incidents. It is the most significant novelty introduced by the rule. The subpart describes in detail the requirements for each step of this HARPC.

In the hazard analysis for human food, there are specific provisions for ready-to-eat food, which is considered is a separate category. In PCAF, all animal food is considered ready to eat.

The hazard analysis and validation of human food must include allergens and allergen cross-contaminations, while these are excluded with animal food.

In PCAF, if preventive control is not completely applied to an identified hazard, but the hazard is not relevant for the customer's livestock, then the customer is not required to apply the preventive control. In that case, however, the customer's written assurance must be included in the records.

PCAF §507.51 - *Modified requirements that apply to a facility solely engaged in the storage of unexposed packaged animal food* - is the same as section PCHF §117.206 - *Modified requirements that apply to a facility solely engaged in the storage of unexposed packaged food.*

D. Modified Requirements. The application of preventive controls is risk-based. In accordance with this principle, businesses that produce and sell a limited amount of food are considered qualified facilities and subject to simpler requirements as described in this subpart.

> PCAF §507.51 - *Modified requirements that apply to a facility solely engaged in the storage of unexposed packaged animal food* - is the same as section PCHF §117.206 - *Modified requirements that apply to a facility solely engaged in the storage of unexposed packaged food.*
>
> PCAF § 507.7 - *Requirements that apply to a qualified facility* matches PCHF § 117.201 - *Modified requirements that apply to a qualified facility,* which is in a different section).

E. Withdrawal of a Qualified Facility Exemption. The subpart explains when the FDA can withdraw the exemption for qualified facilities, how the withdrawal process works, and how facilities can appeal the FDA's decision.

> PCAF §507.200 - *Records subject to the requirements of this subpart* is split into two sections in PCHF:
>
> - §117.320 - *Requirements for official review.*
> - §117.325 - *Public disclosure.*

F. Requirements Applying to Records That Must Be Established and Maintained. It describes what type of records food facilities must keep and what their requirements are.

G. Supply-Chain Program. This subpart describes mandatory controls of food facilities on their suppliers, both domestic and foreign. We will talk about this subpart in detail in chapter 6.

II. APPLICABILITY AND EXEMPTIONS

Applicability and exemptions do not apply to the whole rule but to its single subparts, in particular subpart B (cGMP), C (HARPC) and G (supply chain program).

Types of foods and facilities exempt from Subpart C (HARPC) and Subpart G (Supply Chain Program)

Qualified facilities - §117.5 (a). FSMA grants the status of qualified facilities and a simplified process for preventive controls either to very small businesses or to any business that sells a limited amount of food directly to consumers, or to retail food establishments nearby.

Modified facilities are defined as:

- very small businesses, where a rolling annual average value of human food sold in the last three years adjusted for inflation is less than $1 million. The calculation includes the market value of human food manufactured, processed, packed, or held without sale, or
- facilities with both of the following requisites:
  o the average annual monetary value of all of the sold food that was manufactured, processed, packed or held during the three years prior to the current calendar year - adjusted for inflation - is less $500,000;

o   the value of food sold to *qualified end-users* is higher than the value of the food sold to other businesses.

PCAF §507.1- *Very small business in relation to PCAF means, for purposes of this part, a business (including any subsidiaries and affiliates) averaging less than $2,500,000, adjusted for inflation, per year, during the 3-year period preceding the applicable calendar year in sales of animal food plus the market value of animal food manufactured, processed, packed, or held without sale (e.g., held for a fee or supplied to a farm without sale).*

A *qualified end-user* is either:

- a private individual who resides at any distance from the qualified facility, or
- a retail food establishment located in the same State or Indian reservation of the qualified facility, or within 275 miles.

Fish and fish-based food (CFR 21 part 123) and *juices* (CFR 21 part 120) - §117.5 (b) and *(c)*. These operations will be subject to Hazard Analysis and Critical Control Points (HACCP). However, they still must meet the requirements of cGMP and maintenance of record (subparts B, and F).

Thermally Processed Low-Acid Canned Foods - §117.5 (d), when the facility is required to comply and complies with CFR21 part 113. In this case, the exemption only applies to microbiological risks, while all other hazards will still be subject to HARPC. Low-acid is defined as any foods, other than alcoholic beverages, with a pH above 4.6.

Manufacturing, packaging, labelling, or holding of dietary supplements - §117.5 (e). These facilities are regulated in 21 CFR part 111).

Farms - §117.5 (f). They are required to comply with Standards for Produce Safety (section 419 Federal Food, Drugs and Cosmetics Act) and the Product Safety rule.

Alcoholic beverages - §117.5 (i) are exempt whenever the facility is legally required to have a permit and be registered under section 415 of the Federal Food, Drug and Cosmetics Act, and is subject to the Alcohol and Tobacco Tax and Trade Bureau (TTB).

The exemption also applies to producers of alcoholic beverages that process other types of food, if it is pre-packaged and constitutes less than 5% of the sales of the facility.

§117.5 (j) Facilities that simply store RACs for further processing or distribution. Fruits and vegetables, however, are not exempt. For example, a distributor who buys bags of raw peanuts from farmers and stores them will not be subject to preventive controls. By contrast, a distributor of lettuce and tomatoes will be subject to preventive controls even if they simply store them.

117.7 (a) Facilities that only store packaged food that is not exposed to the environment. However, if the food is time- and temperature-sensitive, it will be subject to the modified requirements of subpart D. Examples of these types of exemptions are fresh-cut fruits and vegetables, fresh herb-infused oils, cream-filled pastries and vitamins, minerals, and dietary ingredients.

The last two exemptions are similar, in that they both involve raw fruits and vegetables. What makes the difference is whether they are packaged or not. Unpackaged fruits and vegetables will be subject to preventive controls, while packaged fruits and vegetables will be subject to modified requirements (along with other foods that are also time- and temperature-sensitive).

Small or very small farm mixed-type facilities -117.5 (g) and (h) are exempt from subpart C and G, and *very small businesses* are also exempt from subpart D (modified requirements) for certain low-risk food/activity combinations, on two conditions:

- such activities are conducted on-farm;
- they would be the only activities subject to the Preventive Controls rule.

There are two types of activity that are part of these low-risk combinations: packing or holding and manufacturing/processing.

The combinations where the activity is packing or holding include, but are not limited to, weighing, conveying or sorting of cocoa products, baked goods or jams. The full list of foods making up these combinations can be found at §117.5 (g)(3).

The combinations where the activity is manufacturing/processing include slicing baked goods, pitting dried plums, or grinding grains. The full list of foods making up these combinations can be found at §117.5 (h)(3).

A few considerations to add about this exemption:

- *§117.5 (g)(2)* from *(i)* to *(x)* specifies the exact meaning of certain food categories in parts (g)(3) and (h)(3). (for example, *'Other fruit and vegetable products'* and *'Processed seeds for direct consumption'*.)
- The list of food categories in (g)(3) and (h)(3) do not include drying/dehydrating of RACs, because these are part of the 'farm' definition and therefore already excluded.
- The size criteria to determine small and very small farms and facilities are the same as outlined in chapter 2.

Types of foods and facilities exempt from Subpart B (current Good Manufacturing Practices)

Current Good Manufacturing Practices do not apply to the following entities - §117.5 (k) - unless this qualification for exemption has been formally withdrawn by the FDA as set out by the rules in subpart E:

- Farms (not mixed type farms)
- Fishing vessels that are not subject to the registration requirements
- Establishments solely engaged in the holding and/ or transportation of one or more raw agricultural commodities

Farm mixed-type facilities are exempt from cGMP for the activities under the 'farm' definition. They are also exempt if the processing activities are limited to hulling, shelling, drying, packing, and/or holding nuts, without additional manufacturing/processing (such as roasting).

Finally, if a farm or a farm mixed-type facility dries or dehydrates RACs that are defined as 'produce' in the produce safety rule (§112.1) it can choose whether to follow cGMP or the Product safety Rule for the part regarding packing and holding of those RACs.

III. CURRENT GOOD MANUFACTURING PRACTICES

FSMA's update of cGMP

The purpose of Current Good Manufacturing Practices (cGMP) is to establish basic operational and environmental conditions for food safety in processing facilities.

cGMP was first introduced in 1969 and then significantly updated before being included in FSMA in Sept 2015 as part of the PC rules. (the last revision before that was in 1986.)

Although the update did not really change cGMP's basic principles, it brought significant additions:

- More detailed descriptions of existing practices
- Addition of parts on allergens control and environmental monitoring for microbial testing
- The word "should" was eliminated to avoid any reference to possible non-binding language
- Training became mandatory

The last change was the most substantial one and was prompted by the very high correlation between food safety incidents and lack of staff training. Under FSMA, **all** personnel handling food - including seasonal employees and contractors - must receive appropriate training. The facility will have to document the content of the training, who received it and when.

'Appropriate' also means that those in charge of overseeing the HARPC process or to conduct audits must receive specific training or have a level of experience recognised as adequate by the FDA.

The different sections of cGMP

Here below is a summary of the nine sections of Current Good Manufacturing Practices. Rather than paraphrasing them, we will give a summary of the main aspects.

Personnel. Includes practices that staff must follow in order to maintain high levels of hygiene and cleanliness, such as the use of nets and gloves, hand washing, plus additional precautions for allergen contaminations. It also includes practices to prevent personnel from contaminating food when they get sick.

Grounds. Areas located outside the facility (roads, yards, and parking lots) must be kept clean and tidy, with special attention given to avoiding pests and dirt coming from neighbours, especially when they are not from other food companies subject to the same rules.

Plant design. The design of the plant must facilitate sanitary operations, providing separate areas to minimise the risk of cross allergen contamination, adequate drainage, lighting and ventilation with screens against pests and insects.

Equipment and utensils. Tools and utensils must be easy to clean (with smooth surfaces and no crevices) and be designed in such a way as to avoid cross-contamination with allergens, lubricants, objects, contaminated water, etc. Food-contact surfaces must be built with non-toxic materials and be resistant to cleaning agents, corrosion and other environmental factors such as sunlight.

Sanitary operations. While the previous sections set out the conditions to create optimal hygienic standards, the part on sanitary operations describes the daily activities to maintain these standards:

- Maintain proper sanitation of surfaces, portable equipment and utensils for both food contact and non-food contact surfaces
- Prevent contamination between non-food- and food-contact materials
- Keep toxic cleaning agents in separate storage. Pesticides must be used only when necessary
- Prevent allergen cross-contamination, paying special attention to movable equipment
- Ensure frequent sanitation of wet processing surfaces, before any use and after any interruption
- Keep low moisture processing surfaces clean and dry
- Use, store, and dispose of single-serve materials appropriately

Sanitary facilities. While sanitary operations remove dirt and sanitise, appropriate design of sanitary facilities ensures that this dirt is effectively removed from the factory floor. Facilities must ensure that:

- Sewage is disposed of directly into the drains, or at least very close to them
- Toilet facilities do not open directly into the processing area

- Location and number of hand-washing facilities are adequate. The same applies to rubbish collection and disposal

Processes and controls. This section is dedicated to all plant operations. In particular:

- General operations: sanitation level, quality control, testing and treatment of contaminated food
- Storing and treatment of raw materials
- Food manufacturing operations

Warehousing and distribution. This is a brief section about how food must be stored and transported in such a way as to avoid all types of adulteration and contamination.

Holding and distribution of human food by-products for use as animal food. It contains details on how to avoid contamination of human food by-products that will be used as animal food.

Define action levels. It includes general provisions about minimising quality defects. It also makes clear that mixing adulterated food with other food to lower the concentration of contaminants is explicitly prohibited, regardless of the final level of adulteration.

IV. THE FOOD SAFETY PLAN AND THE HARPC PROCESS

Compared to HACCP, the Hazard Analysis and Risk-based Preventive Controls is a more holistic, comprehensive and prevention-oriented approach to food safety.

One of the main differences between the two is the expanded scope of preventive controls. In HACCP, a thorough (Prerequisite Program) PRP can lead to mitigation of food safety hazards and hence reduce the need of CCPs. The problem with this model is that it is based on the assumption that the PRP is always applied, although (unlike CCPs), it is not subject to monitoring and verifications.

To solve this failure point, the FDA gave food safety-related PRPs the same importance as CCPs and renamed then preventive controls. Allergen cross-contamination for example, would be part of PRP in HACCP, and not necessarily subject to monitoring. In the HARPC approach however, it would be part of Preventive Controls.

The food safety plan

The foundation of HARPC starts with the food safety plan, where the whole process is described in detail. Although the FDA is flexible about its format, there are a few requirements to follow:

1. It must contain the following parts:

    a. Hazard analysis
    b. Preventive controls
    c. Supply-chain program
    d. Recall plan
    e. Monitoring
    f. Corrective actions
    g. Verification

2. All of them must be written and included in the official records.

3. It must be prepared (or at least its preparation be overseen) by one or more preventive controls qualified individual(s) (PCQI). Their role will be essential in other parts of the food safety plan management, like validating preventive controls, reviewing records and providing justifications for missed timeframes. We will describe PCQI in more detail in chapter 15 of this book.

4. It must be reanalysed whenever:

   a. There is a significant change at the facility that may create the risk of new hazards (or increase the risk of existing ones)
   b. New information on potential hazards becomes available
   c. There is an unanticipated food safety problem
   d. Validation and verification procedures find out that the food safety plan (or parts of it) was ineffective
   e. at least once every three years, if none of the events above occurs

The HARPC process can be broadly divided into two phases: hazard analysis and preventive controls, and preventive controls management.

Hazard analysis and preventive controls

This is a preliminary phase to put the HARPC program in place. It is divided into four steps:

1. Hazard analysis
2. Risk assessment
3. Preventive controls
4. Parameters and values

Hazard analysis. Its purpose is to identify hazards that are "known or reasonably foreseeable." Like in HACCP, hazards can be microbiological, chemical and physical. However, HARPC includes radiological hazards (as part of chemical hazards), allergen control and economically motivated adulteration. The result of the analysis must be recorded in writing when the response is that there are no foreseeable hazards.

The first step is to collect information on all aspects of the facility:

- What food enters the facility (this applies to both raw and processed food)
- The design of the facility and traffic patterns
- All types of operations (transportation, storing, manufacturing, packaging and labelling)
- All tools and machines in use

The list of possible hazards must be based on multiple sources of reliable data (like updated statistics on food safety incidents and scientific literature) other than experience. Here below is a list of reliable sources of information (both free and paid) to conduct a hazard analysis:

- Horizon Scan: https://horizon-scan.fera.co.uk/
- Food Fraud Database on Trello:
  https://www.youtube.com/watch?v=9iaGYD1mDKk
- World bank:
  https://www.youtube.com/watch?v=lAXIrBIS5SQ
- FDA:
  https://www.youtube.com/watch?v=ZY_o0fH2cCs
- CFIA:
  https://www.youtube.com/watch?v=WAOQkdtdFIE

- RASFF:
  https://www.youtube.com/watch?v=8HIB2ATZo1s
- FRANZ:
  https://www.youtube.com/watch?v=d3RVuZ9TaJg

Hazard profiles are not set in stone, but may change throughout the year, so it will be important to use these resources often.

Risk assessment. The next step is to identify those risks that would be of a significant threat for human health and with a high probability to occur in the absence of preventive controls.

Preventive controls. Compared to CCPs, preventive controls are much wider in scope (we will discuss this difference more in detail in part VII of this chapter). Their goal is to significantly minimise or prevent those risks with high probability and severity. The PC rule specifies six areas covered by preventive controls:

1. Processing operations, such as heating, acidification, refrigeration, etc.
2. Allergen cross contamination and mislabelling
3. Sanitation
4. Supply chain
5. Recall plan
6. Other areas including staff training and cGMP

Parameters and values. Each preventive control must have parameters and values indicating the specific safety standard. Any deviation will be considered a red flag. Like for hazard analysis, it is important to base these parameters and values on data from several reliable sources. Here is a list with the most important ones:

- FDA
  - Hazard guides: guidelines, tolerances and action levels - https://www.fda.gov/downloads/Food/GuidanceRegulation/FSMA/UCM517402.pdf
  - Food Code - https://www.fda.gov/Food/GuidanceRegulation/RetailFoodProtection/FoodCode/
  - Pasteurized Milk Ordinance (PMO) - https://www.fda.gov/downloads/food/guidanceregulation/guidancedocumentsregulatoryinformation/milk/ucm513508.pdf
  - Acidified Foods regulations - https://www.fda.gov/Food/GuidanceRegulation/GuidanceDocumentsRegulatoryInformation/AcidifiedLACF/default.htm
- Other regulatory guidelines
  - State and local regulations, tolerances and action levels
  - USDA regulations, tolerances and action levels
- Experts (internal and external): process authorities, university food scientists/microbiologists, consultants, equipment manufacturers, sanitarians, trade association
- Scientific studies: in-house experiments, 3rd party challenge studies (universities or contract labs)
- Scientific literature
  - Peer reviewed journals, food science texts, microbiology texts
  - Food Safety Preventive Controls Alliance information

Preventive Controls management

Preventive controls require a systematic management process, which can be divided into:

1. Monitoring
2. Corrective actions and corrections
3. Verification and validation
4. Recall plan

The purpose of *monitoring* is to verify that the facility is actually implementing all of the preventive controls. Monitoring procedures and frequency must be appropriate to each preventive control, and they both need to be included in the food safety plan.

Corrective actions and corrections. FSMA requires facilities to determine in advance the corrections to take in case of food safety incidents. Their goal is to deal with three priorities:

- To identify and correct the problem
- To test all affected food for safety
- To prevent all affected food from entering commerce, if it is not sure that it is safe.

Next to this, a corrective action procedure must be in place which stipulates what corrective actions are being defined for each breach of a preventive control.

Verification and validation.

Although verification and validation are treated together in the rule, they mean two different things: while **validation** is the process used to determine the appropriate critical limits for hazards that require preventive controls, **verification** is the process of checking that the critical limits that have been set are being met on an ongoing basis.

All parts of the food safety plan are subject to verification:

- proper execution of preventive controls
- monitoring
- preventive actions and corrections
- reanalysis.

Only a subset of the preventive controls needs to be validated. The following preventive controls are exempt from validation and verification alone is sufficient:

- allergen controls
- sanitation controls
- recall plan
- supply chain plan
- other preventive controls for which a written justification is in place

Validation of preventive controls requires several activities:

- Product testing and environmental monitoring
- Review of all written records
- Calibration of all measurement and control devices, with correct maintenance of calibration records from the manufacturer, external calibration agencies or internal activities.

The goal of validation is to ensure that preventive controls are appropriate for the hazard and the facility. It must be conducted or overseen by a qualified individual and completed within a specific timeframe:

- before the food safety plan is implemented, or

- within 90 days after food production has started, or
- within a reasonable timeframe neither deadline can be met. In this case, the justification for this delay must be included in the written records

Recall plan. A recall plan is mandatory for all food hazards requiring preventive controls. It must specify the steps to take in case of food recall, and who is responsible for each one of them. FSMA identifies four main steps in a food recall:

1. Notify and instruct the consignees of the food
2. Notify the public, if appropriate to protect public health
3. Verify that the recall is carried out
4. Dispose of the recalled food. Destroying it is not the only option; the facility could also reprocess or re-direct it or use it in a way that does not represent a safety concern.

The recall procedure can be divided in 5 steps.

Step 1: Establish the recall team members and their responsibilities, such as:

- Decision making. It could be the entire team (by unanimity or majority of opinions) or a specific person (owner, MD)
- Quality Assurance Technical Advisory, to define the details of the food safety issue.
- Media Communication, to inform the general public
- Complaint Investigation, when the food safety incident first originates from a complaint
- Contacting customers who received or may have received the contaminated food

- Contacting the relevant regulatory body (FDA, FSIS or CFIA) and certification body (BRC, IFS, FSSC22000, SQF)
- Legal Counsel, whether in-house or a food lawyer

Step 2: Conduct the complaint investigation (the same procedure applies to issues originated internally), gathering all possible information on:

- The person who made the complaint (name, address, telephone numbers, any illness or injury)
- The problem with the product (allergic reaction, illness, object in the product, chemical taste, etc.)
- The product name, lot code or production date, package type and size, other identifying codes, and a sample of the product if available.
- The name and address of the store where the product was purchased and the date of purchase
- How the complainant stored and handled the product
- The illness caused by the product (when the product was consumed, how many persons are ill, their ages, etc.)
- Whether the complaint was referred to anyone else (This could be Public Health, FDA, CFIA, FSIS, etc.)
- All the findings regarding the complaint

Step 3: Prepare a recall contact lists of people and organisations you may have to inform:

- Names, email, website and phone numbers of the appropriate regulatory agencies and certifying bodies
- Names, email and phone numbers of all customers

- Names and email of relevant trade associations & consumer associations
- Names, email and phone numbers of all potential service providers during a recall:
- Laboratories for microbiological, chemical and physical testing
- Experts (FARRP, Allergen Bureau)
- Law firms
- Insurance companies

Facilities that are involved in a lot of international business may need to inform multiple authorities. Two reliable sources to find them are:

Codex Alimentarius: http://www.fao.org/fao-who-codexalimentarius/about-codex/members/en/
Wikipedia: https://en.wikipedia.org/wiki/List_of_food_safety_organisations

Step 4: Create / update and implement the food recall procedure

- Identify the concern and assemble the recall team
- Notify your applicable regulatory agencies and certification bodies
- Identify all products to be recalled
- Segregate (put on hold) affected products that are under your control
- Prepare a distribution list to trace where the products were shipped
- Prepare a press release (if necessary)
- Notify customers/distributors to inform them on what to do with the recalled products

- Control recalled products that came back to your facility and decide what to do with them
- Decide whether to reprocess, rework, divert or dispose of recalled products
- Perform and effectiveness check (step 5)
- Investigate and fix the root cause of the recall

Step 5: Effectiveness Check

- Perform a mass balance of all product involved, calculating:
  - The total quantity of affected product produced
  - The quantity that is still under your control
  - The returned products from customers / consumers
  - The amount already consumed / not returned from customers (most likely you will have to rely on a good estimate of this amount)

- Confirm recall details and designation of all products with all customers (the most effective way is to call them directly) and ask for proof.
- Keep records of all the details, including shipment documentation and additional photos, which may be important for insurance claims or other legal uses.

Exemptions from preventive controls

In principle, preventive controls must be conducted by the processing facility. However, FSMA allows for some flexibility on this aspect, allowing the food manufacturer / processor to sell food without performing a preventive control, when:

1. the preventive control is a mandatory step in making the food edible. For cocoa beans for example, roasting is both a preventive control and a processing activity, so it will not be listed as a preventive control
2. the preventive control will be performed by the customer the food was shipped to
3. another entity further down the distribution line will perform that control.

The fundamental requirement of these exemptions is that they must be written. The processing facility must specify in the records that the food is "not processed to control the identified hazard" and obtain written assurance from the customer (or the customer's customer) that they will perform that control. This written assurance must be renewed every year.

For this part of written customers provisions, the FDA extended the compliance deadline by two years, in addition to the original compliance date for preventive controls. For example, small businesses with a compliance dated 18 September 2017 will have until 18 September 2019 to comply with the customers written provisions.

V. RECORD KEEPING

Facilities must keep three types of records:

1. *Records, that demonstrate the effective application of food safety preventive controls by the supplier, prior to the "receiving facility." (we will look at them in detail in chapter 6)*

2. Records that demonstrate the application of the facility's food safety plan. These must include the following parts:

- Monitoring of preventive controls
- Corrective actions
- Validation of preventive controls
- Verification of monitoring and corrective actions
- Calibration of process monitoring and verification instruments
- Product testing
- Environmental monitoring
- Records review
- Reanalysis
- Records that document the supply chain program
- Records that document the training of the preventive control qualified individual and the qualified auditor

3. *Records that demonstrate that an identified hazard is being controlled by the customer of the receiving facility, or by entities beyond the first customer.*

Whenever the food is sold without a preventive control and the facility relies on its first customer to apply it, then the facility must include it in the records:

- a disclosure in the shipping documents accompanying the food that the product is not processed to control identified hazards.
- an annual written assurance that the customer has established and is following procedures that will significantly minimize or prevent the identified hazard. A description of such procedures must also be included in the written assurance.

If the manufacturer/processor relies on an entity further down the distribution chain, to control the identified hazard, then the facility must include it in the records:

- A disclosure in the shipping documents accompanying the food to be shipped to the first customer that the product is not processed to control identified hazards;
- An annual written assurance from the first customer that it will disclose in its shipping documents to its customer that the food is not processed to control identified hazards;
- That the customer will sell only to another entity that agrees, in writing, to follow procedures (identified in the written assurance) that will significantly minimize or prevent the identified hazard.

Record requirements

As for their general requirements, records must be:

- kept as original records, true copies, or electronic records
- truthful, accurate, indelible, and legible
- created in real time, and not after the documented activity is performed
- as detailed as necessary

Regarding their content, they must include:

- Adequate information to identify the plant or facility
- The date and - when appropriate - time of the activity documented

- The signature or initials of the person performing the activity
- When appropriate, the identity of the product and lot code

The food safety plan must also include the signature of the owner, operator, or agent in charge of the facility must sign and date the food safety plan, when it is first prepared and every time it is modified

Record retention

- Here are the most important aspects regarding record retention:
- All records must be retained for at least two years from the date they were prepared, even when they are related to discontinued practices or dismissed equipment.
- Records related to qualified facilities must be retained for as long as necessary to support the status of a facility as a qualified facility.
- Records can be stored off-site, except for the food safety plan, which must be kept on-site. Off-site records however, must be retrievable within 24 hours if requested by authorities.
- Electronic records must be accessible from the location to be considered on-site.
- If the facility is closed for a prolonged period, the food safety plan may be transferred to some other accessible location but must be able to be returned to the plant or facility within 24 hours for official review upon request.

VI. MODIFIED REQUIREMENTS

Two types of facilities are subject to modified requirements: qualified facilities and facilities that only store unexposed packaged food.

Qualified facilities

Qualified facilities (see definition in part II of this chapter) are exempt from keeping a written food safety plan, and from following the supply chain verification program.

Although they must implement HARPC, it would be sufficient to self-certify that the facility identified hazards, implemented preventive controls and is monitoring and verifying them.

Alternatively, the qualified facility can self-certify that it is compliant with other non-federal food safety law regulations. This attestation must be accompanied by relevant documentation.

There is no minimum retention period for these records: a qualified facility will have to keep them for as long as necessary to support its status.

How to obtain the status of qualified facility

Businesses that want to receive the status of qualified facilities must submit all supporting documentation to the FDA within specific timeframes, depending on their situation:

- Facilities that are already operational before 17 Sept 2018 will have to submit their requests by the end of 2018

- Facilities that are not operational by 17 Sept 2018, will have to submit their request before starting operations
- Facilities that are already operating as a "not a qualified facility" and want to obtain qualified facility status must submit documentation by the 31st of July of the applicable calendar year.

Beginning in 2020, the qualified facility status must be renewed every 2 years during the period beginning on October 1st and ending on December 31st.

Withdrawal of qualified facility status

The FDA may withdraw qualified facility status following a foodborne illness outbreak.

Before deciding on a withdrawal, the FDA may use other actions such as warning letters, recalls, administrative detentions, etc. and consider the corrective actions of the owner.

The withdrawal of the status follows a specific procedure that is explained in detail in subpart E of the preventive controls rule.

Facilities that only store unexposed packaged food

Facilities that only store unexposed packaged food will have to implement preventive controls only when they also store food that is time- and temperature-sensitive. The implementation of these modified requirements includes all the parts of the standard HARPC process, but it is simplified in that it will only involve the aspect of temperature control.

Modified requirements for these facilities will involve three aspects:

Preventive controls:

- Establishing and implementing preventive controls to minimise or prevent the growth of toxins or pathogens
- Monitoring their implementation with adequate frequency
- Calibrating and monitoring measuring devices.
- Reviewing calibration and monitoring records

In the case of loss of temperature that may create food safety issues, they must:

- Take corrective actions
- Evaluate the safety of affected food
- Prevent affected food from entering commerce, if they cannot ensure it is safe

Record keeping:

- Monitoring
- Corrective actions
- Verification activities

VII. IMPLEMENTING HARPC FROM HACCP

Depending on the situation, a processing facility may have to implement HARPC from scratch or starting from an existing HACCP program.

When building HARPC from scratch, the FDA provides the options to use a Food Safety Plan Builder. Although it does

not guarantee compliance, it is still quite useful because it includes all of the different parts of the food safety plan.

- Builder download: https://www.accessdata.fda.gov/scripts/foodSafetyPlanBuilder/
- Trainingontool:https://www.youtube.com/playlist?list=PLey4Qe-Uxcxb9AGNwFj-oGlquHDZ-tkqo

When the starting point is an existing HACCP program, then HARPC implementation will be divided in two steps:

1. Implementing the additional elements
2. Adapting the existing HACCP through a decision tree

Implementing the additional elements

HARPC is an expanded version of HACCP, so once the adaptation is complete, it is necessary to include the parts that are specific to HARPC.

1. Change nomenclature:
   - From *critical control points* to *preventive controls*
   - From *critical limits* to *parameters and values*

2. Include radiological hazards in the hazard analysis. In particular, facilities may have to:
   - Obtain supporting documentation about whether or not their water supply is at risk
   - Take extra care with any supply from Ukraine or Japan or materials which might otherwise be radioactive or irradiated

3. Include other aspects in the preventive controls:
   - Suppliers
   - allergen cross-contamination control
   - sanitation

4. Implement all the other parts of the food safety plan (monitoring, corrective actions, etc.)

Adapting the existing HACCP through a decision tree

The most effective way to adapt an existing HACCP program is to do a complete reassessment to have a clear idea of all CCPs, PRP and oPRP.

We recommend using the following decision tree

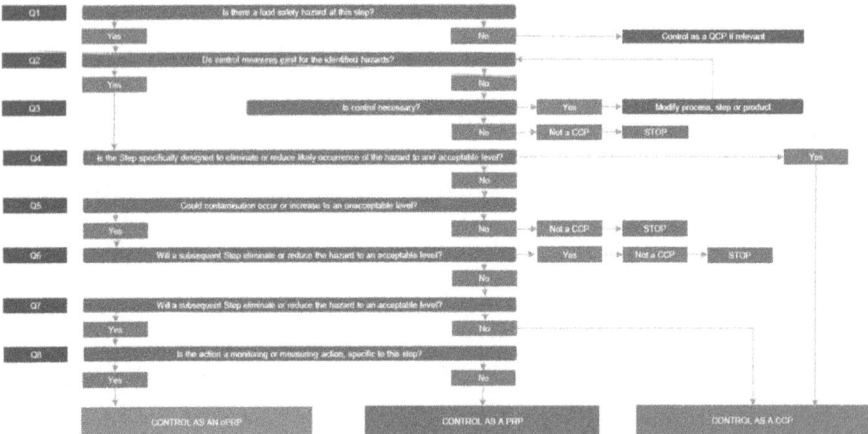

Q1:Is there a food safety hazard at this step?

> If the answer is No, then it you may decide to control it as a Quality Control Point if relevant.

> If the answer is Yes, then proceed to questions 2 and 3.

Q2 and Q3: Do control measures exist for the identified hazard, and is a control necessary?

> If the answer is No to both questions, it means this is not a CCP and the analysis is complete.

If there are no control measures, but control is necessary, then you will have to create them by modifying the process, the step or the product.

If there are already control measures in place (or once you have created them), proceed to Q4.

Q4: Is the Step specifically designed to eliminate or reduce the likely occurrence of the hazard to an acceptable level?

If the answer is Yes, then this step should be considered a CCP, and the analysis is complete.

If the Step is not designed to reduce risk, then proceed to Q5.

Q5: Could contamination occur, or increase to an unacceptable level?

If the answer is No, it means there is no relevant risk for that hazard, and it is not a CCP.

If the answer is Yes, then proceed to question 6.

Q6: Will a subsequent Step eliminate or reduce the hazard to an acceptable level?

If the answer Yes, then this is not a CCP and the analysis is complete.

If the answer is No, then proceed to Q7.

Q7: Is the hazard addressed under Preventive Controls in general?

If the answer is No, then it should be a CCP.

If the answer is Yes, proceed to the last question.

Q8: Is the action a monitoring or measuring action, specific to this step?

If the answer is No, then you can control is as a PRP. If the answer is Yes, then it should be considered an oPRP.

The final step will be to include CCPs, oPRPs and PRPs in the food safety plan as preventive controls.

As a service to the reader we have created an Excel file containing all the hyperlinks which are mentioned in the book. You can download the Excel file via this link: https://www.foodsafety-experts.com/fsma-book-link/

Alternatively, you can also scan this QR code:

CHAPTER 5

Implementation for Plan Pre-ventive Controls for Human and Animal Food

This chapter contains a table which you can use to plan the detailed steps to take towards compliance with the Preventive Controls for Human Food and the Preventive Controls for Animal Food Rules.

The first column of the table identifies the company size, as not all actions are required for all types of companies. Please note that there is a difference in the definition of very small company in relation to Human Food and Animal Food: the first has a threshold of $1,000,000 average sales per year over the last 3 years, and the latter has a threshold of $2,5000,000 average sales per year over the last 3 years.

The second column provides the action to take towards compliance with these FSMA rules.

In the third column you can evaluate whether the action is relevant for your company, based on its size and the current status of FSMA compliance.

In the fourth column you can insert the action you are going to take, but before doing so – please read column five as well, as it contains valuable remarks in relation to the action to take.

In the last three columns you can assign actions to various people in your organization, includ-ing a deadline and a status update for regular review.

The table has been rotated by 90 degrees, so it maximizes the use of the paper and it allows you to make copies more easily. You can also download this table in an Excel file via this link: https://www.foodsafety-experts.com/fsma-book-excel/ . Alternatively, you can scan this QR-code:

Company Size	Item description	Relevant	Action	Remarks	Responsible	Due Date	Status
All	Check FDA registration - Does your facility manufacture, process, pack, or hold food? Then need to register unless exempt (Alcoholic beverages and food produced at same facility so long as it is in prepackaged form and constitutes less than 5% overall sales, Pasteurized Milk Ordinance Regulated Facilities, Retail, Restaurants, USDA, Seafood HACCP, Juice HACCP)			"See https://www.fda.gov/Food/GuidanceRegulation/FoodFacilityRegistration/default.htm https://www.registrarcorp.com/fda-food/"			
All	If your company has a GFSI certification, evalutate the benefits of getting additional certification connected to the GFSI scheme for FSMA complaince			See section of chapter 2 for more details			
All	Create stakeholder management plan			Create a list of stakeholders and decide what actions you need to take involve the important stakeholders.			
All	Create the high level implementation plan			After reading the relevant chapters for your organization, you take all the relevant actionlists and combine these into a single plan. This way you will get a good indication of the overall timing of your implementation project.			
All	Create presentation for senior management to gain buy in and approval						
All	Update your HACCP plan(s) to include additional hazards (radiological), new nomenclature (preventive controls), adjusted decision tree and food fraud aspects			See section 4 and 7 of chapter 4 for more details			
All	Evaluate whether or not to use the Food Defense Plan Builder for replacing the HACCP plan entirely			"Builder download: https://www.accessdata.fda.gov/scripts/foodSafetyPlanBuilder/ Training on tool: https://www.youtube.com/playlist?list=PLey4Qe-Uxcb9AGNwFj-oGIquHDZ-tkqo"			

Company Size	Item description	Relevant	Action	Remarks	Responsible	Due Date	Status
All	Update your recall management procedure			See section 4 of chapter 4 for more details			
All	Update your calibration procedures and checklists			See section 4 of chapter 4 for more details			
All	Update your record retention policy			See section 5 of chapter 4 for more details			
All	Perform supplier risk assessment and determine supplier verification activities			See section 2 of chapter 6 for more details			
All	Determine whether your qualified individual needs formal, FDA approved training or document that the person is qualified based on experience, training and education received in the past.						
All	Check FDA registration - Does your facility manufacture, process, pack, or hold food? Then you need to register unless exempt (Alcoholic beverages and food produced at same facility so long as it is in prepackaged form and constitutes less than 5% overall sales, Pasteurized Milk Ordinance Regulated Facilities, Retail, Restaurants, USDA, Seafood HACCP, Juice HACCP)			"See https://www.fda.gov/ Food/GuidanceRegulation/ FoodFacilityRegistration/default.htm https://www.registrarcorp.com/fda-food/"			
Large	Check the required changes in relation to current Good Manufacturing Practices and create separate actions for each gap			See section 3 of chapter 4 for more details			
Small	Check the required changes in relation to current Good Manufacturing Practices and create separate actions for each gap			See section 3 of chapter 4 for more details and/ or use the Small Company Compliance Guideline of the FDA			
Very Small	Check the required changes in relation to current Good Manufacturing Practices and create separate actions for each gap			See section 3 of chapter 4 for more details and/ or use the Small Company Compliance Guideline of the FDA			

CHAPTER 6

The Supply Chain Program and the Foreign Supplier Verification Program

I. JOINING THE LINKS OF A BROKEN SUPPLY CHAIN

In the phrase 'food supply chain', the true extent of the word 'chain' is not always fully appreciated. And yet, it is exactly in the complex web of passages (see chapter 1 for a visual representation) from one processing, storing or labelling facility to the other, that many food contaminations happen and get out of control.

One of the goals of FSMA is to strengthen the connections between each link of the food supply chain, by making food facilities responsible for the level of compliance of their suppliers, whether they are from the US or not. For foreign suppliers it means that, even if they are compliant with their local food safety laws, they may have to implement several FSMA provisions and document them, if they want to enter the US food market.

The principles of supply chain controls and typical scenarios

FSMA regulates supply chain controls in two sections: The Risk-based Supply-chain Program in subpart G of the Preventive Controls rule, and the Foreign Supply Verification Program, which is a rule on its own. The FSVP rule regulates the supply chain program that US companies must follow with foreign suppliers. It came into effect not long after the Preventive Controls rule, and is based on the same provisions, with the addition of specific checks.

Under FSMA's definitions, there are three entities involved in the supply chain.

The receiving facility is a food processing or manufacturing facility that is subject to subpart C on HARPC of the Preventive Controls rule.

The food importer is a US-based owner or consignee of an article of food. Alternatively, it can be the US agent or representative of the foreign owner or consignee of that food, as confirmed in a signed statement of consent.

The supplier is the last establishment - before the receiving facility - that either grew or processed the food or raised the animal. It is not necessarily the one that shipped the ingredients: if the shipping facility just performed minimal activities like labelling, it would not be considered a supplier.

In very broad terms, receiving facilities are subject to the provisions in subpart G, while importers are subject to the FSVP rule. This distinction, however, is merely conceptual and does not always identify two different categories: a receiving facility that buys raw materials or other ingredients directly from foreign suppliers is also considered an importer, so it will be subject to FSVP.

We can therefore have three scenarios where either part is applicable:

1. *The receiving facility is subject to HARPC and buys raw materials or other ingredients from a domestic supplier.* In this case, the facility will implement supply chain controls following subpart G. We will discuss the requirements in part II of this chapter.

2. *The receiving facility is subject to HARPC and buys raw materials or other ingredients from a foreign supplier.* If the facility is also sourcing ingredients from domestic suppliers and is compliant with the requirements of subpart G of the Preventive Controls rule, it will be compliant with most requirements of FSVP by simply applying the same practices to foreign suppliers. There will be, however, specific additional requirements. If the facility only sources from foreign suppliers, then the FSVP rule will be the only reference. We will discuss the additional requirements of the FSVP rule in part III of this chapter.

3. *A food importer that is not subject to the Preventive Controls rule* must follow the FSVP rule.

On their end, both domestic and foreign suppliers must be aware of the provisions in subpart G, so they can be aware of what is expected from them if they want to be approved by receiving facilities and importers.

Qualified Individuals and Auditors

The supply chain program is part of the food safety plan. Therefore, a Preventive Control Qualified Individual must prepare it or oversee its preparation. Onsite audits require a specific expertise, so they must be conducted by a Qualified Auditor.

One of the required skills of Qualified Individuals and Auditors is their ability to read and understand any relevant food safety record. This is particularly important with foreign suppliers, as it may be necessary to understand documents provided in other languages. (see chapter 14 on Training for further details.)

II. THE RISK-BASED SUPPLY CHAIN PROGRAM

Applicability and exemptions

The supply chain program in subpart G applies to raw materials and other ingredients when they present a hazard that requires a preventive control, which was applied by the supplier or a third entity.

Examples of these other entities could be:

- a non-supplier that also applies controls to certain produce
- a company under different management that performs growing, harvesting, and packing activities
- a broker

By contrast, the supply chain program does not apply when:

- The food is not subject to preventive controls as per §117.5
- The preventive control will be applied by the receiving facility
- The receiving facility will apply a necessary processing step that also acts as a preventive control (e.g. roasting cocoa beans)
- The receiving facility will rely on its customers for the application of the preventive controls, following the requirements on written assurances in §117.136 (see the part on preventive controls exemptions in chapter 4)
- The food is supplied for research and evaluation, provided that:
  - It is not sold or distributed to the public
  - It is supplied in small quantities
  - any unused part is disposed of

The supply chain program is based on the following four activities:

- evaluating and approving suppliers before buying ingredients from them
- conducting and documenting ongoing verification activities
- taking corrective actions whenever necessary
- establishing written procedures and maintaining records.

EVALUATING AND APPROVING SUPPLIERS

Before buying ingredients from any supplier, facilities must evaluate and approve them, and only do business with the approved ones. Evaluation must be repeated every time there is a significant change in the risk profile of the supplier (e.g. ingredients change), the supplier's performance or their internal procedures. If no change happens, re-evaluation must be done at least once every three years.

To approve suppliers, facilities must consider the following two elements.

Hazard analysis and risk assessment of the food. The analysis will consider all the possible hazards coming from each ingredient and then assess the severity and probability of that hazard. The preventive controls that were previously applied and what entity applied them (whether the supplier or third-party) are also included in the analysis. Those hazards with a high severity and probability to occur will be included in the supply chain program.

In real scenarios, there will be a wide range of foreseeable hazards for any given ingredient. For their assessment, facilities can use several sources, both free and paid, to have access to reliable data. Here is a list of the most important ones:

- US Pharmacopeial Convention (USP): https://www.foodfraud.org/
- US National Center for Food Protection and Defense (NCFPD): https://foodprotection.umn.edu/
- US Michigan State University: http://foodfraud.msu.edu/

- Horizon Scan: https://horizon-scan.fera.co.uk
- Food Fraud Database on Trello:
  https://www.youtube.com/watch?v=9iaGYD1mDKk
- World bank:
  https://www.youtube.com/watch?v=lAXIrBIS5SQ
- FDA:
  https://www.youtube.com/watch?v=ZY_o0fH2cCs
- CFIA:
  https://www.youtube.com/watch?v=WAOQkdtdFIE
- RASFF:
  https://www.youtube.com/watch?v=8HIB2ATZo1s
- FRANZ:
  https://www.youtube.com/watch?v=d3RVuZ9TaJg

The supplier's performance. This aspect includes different things such as:

- The procedures and processes the supplier uses to treat those ingredients.
- The supplier's history of compliance with food regulations (warning letters, food recalls, complaints from consumers or customers, etc)
- Their food defence plan.
- The food safety history of the supplier regarding the ingredients, such as the results of tests or audits.
- Any other relevant elements such as storage and transportation practices

Verification activities

Once the facility has evaluated and approved the supplier, its next requirement will be to conduct verification activities on the ingredients before using them, and on an ongoing basis afterwards. The FDA is somewhat flexible regarding what activities to conduct, but provides a list to choose from:

- Onsite audits
- Sampling and testing
- Review of relevant food safety records
- Other activities, depending on the type of ingredient and supplier's performance (e.g. official government controls by the local authorities and proof thereof.)

Verification activities can also be performed by a third party, but not by the supplier itself. Other inappropriate interferences from the supplier would be:

- determining the appropriate verification activities
- providing a review of their own food safety records
- conducting audits

Onsite audits. For certain hazards that the FDA considers particularly serious (identified with the acronym of SAHCODHA, or Serious Adverse Health Consequences or Death to Humans or Animals), FSMA explicitly indicates onsite audits as the appropriate verification activity.

The general requirements for an onsite audit are:

- It must include a review of the supplier's food safety plan and of the implementation of the preventive control for that particular hazard
- It must be conducted before using the ingredient and at least once per year afterwards
- It must be conducted by a qualified auditor (QA)
- The QA can be an employee of the facility or a third-party certification agency, but not someone from the supplier's company

It is not mandatory to conduct an annual onsite audit if:

- there is a written justification that other verification activities and/or less frequent onsite auditing provide adequate levels of control of that hazard
- the supplier has received an inspection from the FDA or other federal or non-federal Agencies within one year from the date the audit should be conducted

When audits are conducted on non-SAHCODHA hazards there is no minimum frequency required.

When preventive controls are applied by an entity other than the supplier, the receiving facility must receive and review the relevant documentation from that entity.

Corrective actions

Whenever a facility finds out that the supplier is not applying the necessary controls to the identified hazards, it must take corrective actions to prevent adulteration of the food and make sure that unsafe food does not enter the market. In this case, the procedures and requirements are the same as those regarding corrective actions in the Preventive Controls rule (§117.150).

Simplified supply chain procedures

With certain very small suppliers, some requirements of the supply chain program are simplified. Such suppliers can be:

- qualified facilities
- farms or mixed-type farm facilities that are not covered by the Produce Safety rules (see chapter 12 for more details)
- shell-egg producers with less than 3,000 laying hens

In this case, the supply chain program is simplified, in that:

- The evaluation of the supplier performance can be limited to their compliance history, with no need to consider processes and practices or their food safety history
- It is not necessary to conduct verification activities, but the facility must obtain form the supplier written assurance that:
  o they qualify for being part of one of those categories. This assurance must be provided before the supplier is approved, and once per year after that
  o they acknowledge that their food is subject to section 402 of the Federal Food, Drug, and Cosmetic Act regarding adulteration or,
  o (if they are a qualified facility) they are compliant with the relevant FDA food safety regulations.

The last two assurances must be provided before the supplier is approved, and once every two years after that.

Written procedures and record keeping

Facilities must keep written records with a description of:

- the supply chain program
- compliance with FSVP (see next section of this chapter)
- procedures for receiving raw materials and ingredients and the documentation to demonstrate their application
- the procedure for suppliers' approval
- determination of verification activities
- onsite audits

- corrective actions taken in response to audits or to any other verification activity
- sampling and testing conducted by the receiving facility
- a supplier's food safety records
- other verification activities, including alternatives to onsite audits
- written assurances from qualified facilities, farms, or egg-shell producers that they are entitled to modified requirements
- relevant documentation from the supplier, such as their own sampling and testing activities
- verification activities conducted by third entities when the preventive control is not applied by the supplier

The general requirements of written records are the same as in subpart F of the Preventive Controls rule (see part on record requirements in chapter 4).

III. THE FOREIGN SUPPLIER VERIFICATION PROGRAM

The FSVP rule extends the supply chain-applied controls to foreign suppliers, to ensure that all the food that comes from abroad has the same safety standards and level of health protection as the one from domestic suppliers.

The standards are those required by the Federal Food, Drug, and Cosmetic Act regarding hazard analysis and risk-based preventive controls for certain foods, produce safety, food adulteration and allergens.

In general, all facilities and businesses that meet the definition of importers must follow the FSVP rule for all types of food. However, certain categories of food or importers are exempt, or subject to modified requirements.

Food exempt from the FSVP

§ 1.501(b). Juice and seafood products that are subject to § 120 and § 123. They are subject to the importation rules of those parts. This even holds true if the company sources other ingredients than juice or seafood, as long as the finished product falls into these respective categories.

§ 1.501(c). Food for research and evaluations. As for subpart G, this type of food cannot be distributed to the public, must be clearly labelled and provide in a quantity consistent with its purpose. Additionally, it must be accompanied by an electronic declaration to US Customs and Border Protection regarding its use.

§ 1.501(d). Food imported for personal consumption. In this case, the buyer must be a private individual and not a business, the quantity must be consistent with personal consumption and the food cannot be distributed to the public.

§ 1.501(e). Alcoholic beverages are exempt if the foreign supplier would have had the same requirements as if they were they operating in the US:

- it would be legally required to have a permit
- it would be legally required to be registered under section 415 of the Federal Food, Drug and Cosmetics Act and is subject to the Alcohol and Tobacco Tax and Trade Bureau (TTB).

However, this simplified procedure only applies to food that will not be further processed, whether it is packaged or not. It does not apply to food that will be used as ingredient for further processing.

IV. THE VOLUNTARY QUALIFIED IMPORTER PROGRAM

Food importers that meet certain requirements can enrol in the FDA's Voluntary Qualified Importer Program.

It is a fee-based program (currently, the fee is about $16,400 per year), which grants faster entry of the food. In most cases, the FDA will not conduct any sample or testing for food covered by the program. However, when samples or tests are necessary (generally because of specific situations, for example an investigation on an outbreak or illness), the Agency will help speed-up importation by:

- examining the food at its destination or another location chosen by the importer, whenever possible
- assisting the importer with exporting the food back to the supplier, in case the entry is denied
- prioritising the analysis of collected samples
- offering a dedicated help desk

Being part of the program also gives importers public recognition, thanks to the publication of their details on the FDA's VQIP web page.

Other than the paying the fee, the requirements to enrol in the program are:

- Implementing a Quality Assurance Program (QAP). The FDA defines it as the "compilation of the written policies and procedures you will use to ensure adequate control over the safety and security of the foods you import." The QAP must contain a description of:

o   the corporate policy related to food safety and security of the supply chain;

o   the management structure;

o   food safety policies and procedures;

o   the food defence system for foods that are subject to the Intentional Adulteration (IA) rule;

o   qualifications of qualified individuals and auditors;

o   procedures that ensure the QAP is implemented;

o   procedures for establishing and maintaining records;

o   definitions used in the QAP;

o   references to information or sources used to develop and implement the QAP

- having a 3+-year history of importing food to the United States
- having a DUNS number
- using paperless filers/brokers who received an acceptable rating during their last FDA Filer Evaluation. In its monitoring and verification activity, the FDA will often have to rely on information provided by non-FDA personnel. The Agency therefore considers the way these individuals operate as very important
- no ongoing FDA administrative or judicial action, or other history of non-compliance with food safety regulations by the importer, other entities in the supply chain, or for the food

- being compliant with FSVP or HACCP regulations
- no history of US Customs and Border Protection penalties, forfeitures, or sanctions related to any imported FDA-regulated product in the last 3 years
- providing certifications issued by FDA's accredited third-parties for each foreign supplier

This last requirement is causing some delays in the implementation of the VQIP. The FDA officially started to accept applications in January 2018 but, given the extra time necessary for the accreditation of third-parties, importers were not able to apply before the end of May 2018.

As a service to the reader we have created an Excel file containing all the hyperlinks which are mentioned in the book. You can download the Excel file via this link: https://www.foodsafety-experts.com/fsma-book-link/

Alternatively, you can also scan this QR code:

CHAPTER 7

Implementation Plan Supplier Management, FSVP and VQIP

This chapter contains a table which you can use to plan the detailed steps to take towards compliance with the Supplier Management aspects of the Preventive Controls for Human Food and the Preventive Controls for Animal Food Rules, the Foreign Supplier Verification Rule and the Voluntary Qualified Importers Program.

The first table in this chapter combines the actions in relation to the Supplier Management aspects of the Preventive Controls for Human Food and the Preventive Controls for Animal Food Rules and the Foreign Supplier Verification Rule. The second table contains all the ac-tions in relation to the Voluntary Qualified Importers Program.

The first column of the table identifies the company size. In this case, the actions apply to all companies, irrespective of size.

The second column provides the action to take towards compliance with these FSMA rules.

In the third column you can evaluate whether the action is relevant for your company, based on the current status of FSMA compliance.

In the fourth column you can insert the action you are going to take, but before doing so – please read column five as well, as it contains valuable remarks in relation to the action to take.

In the last three columns you can assign actions to various people in your organization, includ-ing a deadline and a status update for regular review.

The table has been rotated by 90 degrees, so it maximizes the use of the paper and it allows you to make copies more easily. You can also download this table in an Excel file via this link: https://www.foodsafety-experts.com/fsma-book-excel/ . Alternatively, you can scan this QR-code:

Company Size	Item description	Relevant	Action	Remarks	Responsible	Due Date	Status
All	"Check whether your facility is exempt of the FSVP Rule: - Juice and seafood from foreign suppliers that are in compliance with the respective HACCP regulations (21 CFR part 120 or 123) and ingredients that are used by the importer in the manufacturing or processing of juice and seafood products in accordance with the respective HACCP regulations - Food produced in compliance with FDA's low acid canned food requirements in 21 CFR part 113 (exempt with respect to microbiological hazards controlled by 21 CFR part 113 only) - Alcoholic beverages if supplied by a company that when based in the USA would need to apply for a permit and has an FDA registration number according to the Food, Drug and Cosmetics Act. - Food that is transshipped through the United States or that is imported for future export and not sold or distributed in the United States - Food that is manufactured/processed, raised, or grown in the United States, exported, and returned to the United States without further manufacturing/processing - Meat, poultry, and egg products which are regulated by the USDA at the time of import - You import only from a country with a reconized scheme (currently Australia & New Zealand only)"			"You must document that you are exempt based on the indicated aspects and make sure that you keep track of potential issues at your supplier. You must review your supplier upfront in terms of adherence to PCHF or PCAF rule implementation. In case of issues you must take swift and apt action to resolve this. If food safety related issues occur, and audit within 3 months is still required. Auditing can be delegated to other qualified individuals outside your company as long as the audit report is interpreted by your qualified individual. For full details see appendix 5 of the FSVP Course Participants Manual In all other cases execute all the actions as listed below"			
All	Assess whether all individuals performing activities for the Foreign Supplier Verification Rule are qualified to do so			If necessary follow formal FSVP training (FSPCA approved)			
All	Make sure you as an importer have a DUNS number			See: https://fdadunslookup.com/			

Company Size	Item description	Relevant	Action	Remarks	Responsible	Due Date	Status
All	Plan your foreign supplier audits at least every 3 years and when a serious (food safety related) issue occurs (within 3 months)						
All	"Foreign suppliers from an officially recognized food safety system: - get documentation to verify that the system is officially recognized by the FDA - make sure the supplier is compliant with local legislation before import and thereafter on a continuous basis"						
All	"Check whether your organization complies with all requirements for VQIP: - documented Quality Assurance Program (QAP) - Assurance of compliance with the supplier verification and other importer responsibilities under the applicable FSVP or HACCP regulations - Current facility certification, including farms, issued under FDA's Accredited Third-Party Certification regulations for each foreign supplier of food in VQIP - 3+ year history of importing food to the United States - No ongoing FDA administrative or judicial action, or other history of non-compliance with food safety regulations by the importer, other entities in the supply chain, or for the food - Have a Dun & Bradstreet (D&B) Data Universal Numbering System (DUNS) number"			See section 3 of chapter 6 for more details			
All	"Send in your application via: https://www.fda.gov/Food/GuidanceRegulation/ImportsExports/Importing/ucm490823.htm"						

CHAPTER 8

Intentional Adulteration and Food Defense

I. CLOSING THE CIRCLE ON FOOD SAFETY

In the rule on Mitigation Strategies to Protect Food Against Intentional Adulteration, the FDA - for the first time - made it mandatory for food facilities to develop and implement a food defense plan against intentional adulteration.

The food risk matrix (see chapter 1) divides intentional adulteration in two categories. One is food fraud, or Economically Motivated Adulteration (EMA), where fraudsters adulterate food with cheaper ingredients to decrease its cost or mislabel it to increase its supposed value. The other type is malicious or ideologically motivated adulteration with the intention of causing illness, injury or death to the general public. Examples are a disgruntled employee or terrorists.

Only the latter type is within the scope of the Intentional Adulteration rule, where the purpose of the defense plan is protecting "food from intentional acts of adulteration where there is an intent to cause wide scale public health harm."

By contrast, EMA is addressed in the Preventive Controls rule, where HARPC must also consider hazards that "may be intentionally introduced for purposes of economic gain."

According to the FDA, the reason for this separation is that "addressing economically motivated adulteration worked better under the preventive controls framework, which focuses on hazards that are known or reasonably foreseeable." For a food facility, the risk of food fraud comes mainly from suppliers. With its focus on supply chain control, the Preventive Controls rule can therefore be quite effective in preventing food safety issues caused by food frauds.

However, real-life scenarios are not always that clear-cut. In fact, there may be cases where preventive controls detect or prevent a malicious adulteration, or where mitigation strategies detect or prevent unintentional contaminations.

Although EMA and malicious adulteration have different goals, they're both caused by a voluntary criminal act. That voluntariness may require different types of countermeasures, compared to unintentional or natural food safety issues.

The difference between the food safety and the food defense plans lies exactly in the target of such countermeasures.

While preventive controls focus on food processing activities and sanitation practices, mitigation strategies tend to protect and limit access to food to minimise or eliminate the opportunities for ill-intentioned individuals to contaminate it. Also, while preventive controls are based on scientific data, mitigation strategies rely mainly on statistical data and the study of human motives.

Together, these two types of controls aim to create a 360° protection around food.

II. WHO IT APPLIES TO AND WHO IS EXEMPT

In general, the Intentional Adulteration rule applies to all facilities, whether in the US or abroad, that processes, pack, or hold food for the US market and required to register with the FDA (see chapter 2 for details on registration).

However, certain types of facilities, foods or activities are exempt.

§121.5 (a) Very small businesses (see definition in chapter 1). In this case, however, facilities must provide documentation to prove their very small business status and retain it for 2 years.

§121.5 (b) Facilities whose only activity is to store food. Examples are warehouses, cold storage facilities, storage silos, grain elevators. However, those that store food in liquid form in tanks are subject to the rule.

§121.5 (c) Activities such as packing, re-packing, labelling, or re-labelling of food that comes already pre-packaged where the container that directly contacts the food remains intact.

§121.5 (d) Farming activities subject to the Standards for Produce Safety rule.

§ 121.5 (e) Alcoholic beverages at a facility that:

- is legally required to have a permit and
- is legally required to be registered under section 415 of the Federal Food, Drug and Cosmetics Act and is subject to the Alcohol and Tobacco Tax and Trade Bureau (TTB)

The exemption also applies to foreign facilities that would have the same requirements were they operating in the US.

Facilities with the requirements above are also exempt for food other than alcoholic beverages, if it's pre-packaged in a way to prevent any direct human contact and constitutes no more than 5 percent of the overall sales of the facility.

§ 121.5 (f) Animal food.

§ 121.5 (g) Small or very small farm mixed-type facilities for specific on-farm activities, such as manufacturing, processing, packing or holding of the following foods:

eggs (in-shell, other than raw agricultural commodities, e.g., pasteurized); and

game meats (whole or cut, not ground or shredded, without secondary ingredients).

To be exempt, however, such activities must be the only activities conducted by the business subject to section 418 of the Federal Food, Drug, and Cosmetic Act.

III. DEVELOPING A FOOD DEFENSE PLAN.

The rules on Intentional Adulteration and Preventive Controls use distinct terminology: food defense plan, vulnerabilities and mitigation strategies, as opposed to food safety plan, hazards and preventive controls.

The creation of the food defense plan, however, follows a parallel process:

1. identify critical vulnerabilities
2. decide, implement and monitor mitigation strategies
3. take corrective actions when necessary
4. maintain written records.

The Intentional Adulteration rule requires two levels of qualification for the individuals involved in the food defense plan. The staff in charge of applying mitigation strategies must have an appropriate level of education, training or experience, and an additional training on food defense awareness. The team in charge of preparing the food defense plan must have a qualification based on a standardised FDA curriculum or an equivalent combination of training and experience.

The vulnerability assessment

A vulnerability is a point, step, or procedure that may create the opportunity to commit an act of intentional adulteration.

The written vulnerability assessment must describe the whole process, regardless of the outcome. Its purpose is to identify *significant* vulnerabilities, which are defined as those that could cause a wide-scale harm to public health if exploited.

The difference between a non-significant and a significant vulnerability depends on the answers to three questions:

- How severe and widespread would the impact on public health be, if it were exploited by an attacker?
- Does it offer an easy access point to an attacker?
- Would an attacker have the necessary ability to exploit the vulnerability?

During the assessment, facilities must consider the possibility that the attacker may be external (for example a terrorist acting in name of political or religious beliefs) but also internal, for example a disgruntled employee.

The rule is quite flexible regarding where to look for significant vulnerabilities and what method to use. However, the FDA identified four key activities that repeatedly showed particularly high vulnerability during several assessments, regardless of the type of food.

Bulk liquid receiving and loading. The typical example is the liquid being unloaded after arrival or loaded to be shipped from the facility. In this case there is a high risk because the contaminant could easily be distributed throughout the liquid.

Liquid storage and handling. High-risk for the same reasons of receiving and loading.

Secondary ingredient handling. This is a step where ingredients other than the main one are prepared or mixed together before being added to the preparation. The risk in this case is that a small quantity of contaminant could easily reach the main preparation and increase the scale of the impact.

Mixing and similar activities, like blending, homogenizing, or grinding. This activity is at high-risk because a contaminant, if added, could go unnoticed and blend with the rest of the ingredients.

How to conduct a vulnerability assessment

There are several risk management methods that facilities can follow to conduct a vulnerability assessment. Here we will describe the most common ones.

Threat Assessment Critical Control Points (TACCP)

The TACCP model was developed by The British Standards Institution and modelled on HACCP.

'Threat' in TACCP is defined as "something that can cause loss or harm which arises from the ill-intent of people." Threats can come from any level:

- Upstream: Sabotage of the supply chain leading to disruption and potential shortages
- Inside the facility: Malicious contamination with toxic materials causing ill-health and death
- Downstream: misuse of food and drink products and materials for terrorist or criminal purposes (e.g. extortion)

In general, the goal of TACCP is to answer four key questions:

- Who might want to attack us?
- How might they do it?
- Why are we vulnerable?
- How can we stop them?

The process follows the following workflow:

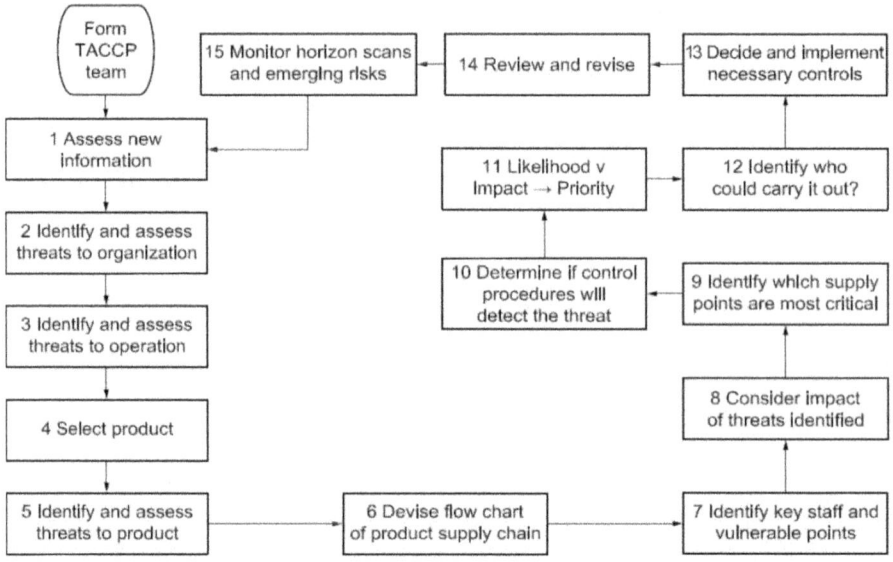

Assemble the team. Because threats may come from anywhere, the food defense team will include individuals from different areas and disciplines such as:

- Security
- HR
- Food technology
- Process engineering
- Production and operations
- Purchasing and supply
- Distribution
- Communications
- Commercial/marketing

Conduct the assessment. The first task of the food defense team will be to examine all new information available on intentional adulteration and focus on possible vulnerabilities of three key elements: the product, the premises, and the organisation. For each element, there are several questions that can be used as a guide. Here we give a few examples.

Threats to products:

- Have there been significant cost increases which have affected this product?
- Does this product have religious, ethical or moral significance for some people?
- Could this product be used as an ingredient in a wide range of popular foods?
- Does the product contain ingredients or other material sourced from overseas?

Threats to premises:

- Are premises located in politically or socially sensitive areas?
- Do premises share access or key services with controversial neighbours?
- Are new recruits appropriately screened?
- Are premises services appropriately screened?
- Are external utilities adequately protected?
- Are hazardous materials which could be valuable to hostile groups stored on site?
- Are large numbers of people using the location?
- Do any employees have reason to feel disgruntled or show signs of dissatisfaction?
- Are internal audit arrangements independent?
- Have key roles been occupied by staff for many years with little supervision?

Threats to the organisation:

- Is the business under foreign ownership by nations involved in international conflict?
- Is there a celebrity or high-profile chief executive or proprietor?
- Is there a reputation of significant links, customer, suppliers etc. with unstable regions of the world?
- Are brands regarded as controversial by some?
- Does the business or customers supply high profile customers or events?

Assessing likelihood and impact. Once vulnerabilities are identified, the next step will be to assess and score the risk that these may be exploited for intentional adulteration and what the impact would be, if that happened. Here, there are a few aspects to consider.

To assess likelihood:

- Would an attacker achieve their goal if successful?
- Would they have access to the product or process?
- Would they be deterred by protective measures?
- Would they prefer other targets?
- Would an attack be detected before it had any impact?

To assess risk:

- How many people would be impacted if contamination would occur
- How severe would the health impact be?
- Would the consequences be illness, serious illness with lasting effects, or death?

The final score will provide a list of significant vulnerabilities to prioritise in the food defense plan.

The CARVER + Shock method

This method has its origins during the Vietnam war, when the US Army Special Forces elaborated the score-based CARVER matrix to evaluate specific targets and better allocate attack resources.

The food industry adapted the offensive nature of the matrix for food defense purposes: with the CARVER plus Shock method, the facility becomes the possible target and tries to think like an attacker would.

CARVER is an acronym for:

- Criticality: the measure of public health and economic impacts of an attack
- Accessibility: the ability to physically access and leave a target
- Recuperability: the ability of a system to recover from an attack
- Vulnerability: the ease of accomplishing the attack
- Effect: the amount of direct loss from an attack measured by loss in production
- Recognizability: the ease of identifying targets

The seventh element is the 'Shock' attribute, which measures the combination of the health, economic, and psychological impacts of an attack.

The attractiveness of each attribute is ranked from 1 to 10, according to precise criteria.

Overall, this method requires the input of a lot of detailed information, for example batch size, serving size and servings per batch. That's one of the reasons why the FDA stepped away from this approach.

SSAFE (PWC + WUR + Industry Partners)

This vulnerability assessment method was developed by the global non-profit organization SSAFE to prevent economically motivated adulteration. However, it can be quite useful to assess vulnerabilities for all types of intentional adulterations.

The assessment tool has both an online and an Excel version and is divided in 6 parts:

1. An initial decision tree to determine what elements need a vulnerability assessment. This could be an ingredient, product, brand, site, country or division.
2. A scoping sheet with the name and roles of the members of the food defense team and the list what elements to assess and why.
3. 50 assessment questions regarding two aspects: the risk of being the target of criminal behaviours from the supply chain, based on opportunities and motivations, and the mitigation strategies currently in place within the company. For each question, the tool provides three possible answers that indicate if the risk of incurring in criminal behaviours or the level of protection are low, moderate or high.
4. Based on the answers, the tool uses spider webs to create a visual representation of the level of risk. In the first set of graphs, opportunities, motivations and controls are presented singularly. The second set groups together opportunities and motivations and selects the level of protection of internal hard controls.
5. An output sheet with the mitigation strategies assigned to the identified vulnerabilities
6. A final report

FDA Food Defense Plan Builder

https://www.fda.gov/Food/FoodDefense/
ToolsEducationalMaterials/ucm349888.htm

The importance of using the right information

The methods we described are all quite different form one another. The principle they all have in common, though, is that to prevent malicious acts of an attacker it's important to think like one.

The first to imagine what a potential criminal would do is to learn what real ones did in real cases, what vulnerabilities they exploited and their motives. There are several reputable sources where a food defense team can get that type of information:

- US Pharmacopeial Convention (USP): https://www.foodfraud.org/
- US National Center for Food Protection and Defense (NCFPD): https://foodprotection.umn.edu/
- US Michigan State University: http://foodfraud.msu.edu/
- Horizon Scan: https://horizon-scan.fera.co.uk/
- Trello: https://www.youtube.com/watch?v=9iaGYD1mDKk
- World bank: https://www.youtube.com/watch?v=lAXIrBIS5SQ
- FDA: https://www.youtube.com/watch?v=ZY_o0fH2cCs
- CFIA: https://www.youtube.com/watch?v=WAOQkdtdFIE

- RASFF: https://www.youtube.com/watch?v=8HIB2ATZo1s
- FRANZ: https://www.youtube.com/watch?v=d3RVuZ9TaJg

Mitigation strategies

The purpose of mitigation strategies is to minimise or eliminate the risk of intentional adulterations. Although there is no particular specification about what mitigation strategies to adopt, they must have the following requirements:

- To be prepared by a qualified individual
- To be risk-based. This means that the food defense plan must prioritise the vulnerabilties with the highest risk of exploitation and the widest potential damage to public health.
- To be consistent with the "current scientific understanding of food defense at the time of the analysis."
- To include a written explanation of why they will be effective. A simple description of the strategy won't be sufficient.

There are many types of mitigation strategies. For example:

- Raw material testing
- Supply chain audits
- Use of tamper evidence on incoming raw materials
- Enhanced supplier approval checks
- Changes to the supply chain

Change to product ingredients

The FDA and the USDA have two databases with many types of mitigation strategies to choose from, which can be a valuable help to food defense teams:

The Food Defense Mitigation Strategies Database (FDA): https://www.accessdata.fda.gov/scripts/ fooddefensemitigationstrategies/

The Food Defense Risk Mitigation Tool (USDA): https://www.fsis.usda.gov/wps/portal/fsis/topics/ food-defense-defense-and-emergency-response/tools-resources-training/risk-mitigation-tool/ct_index

Managing the food defense plan

When significant vulnerabilities are associated to one or more mitigation strategies, they become actionable process steps. The 'action' in this case is the management system, which includes four parts.

Monitoring procedures. A description of the procedure, frequency, and outcome must be included in the food defense plan.

Corrective actions. The plan must include a description of what corrective actions will be taken if the food implementation is not working as intended, and what actions were actually taken.

Verification of the effectiveness every management activity of the food defense plan.

Reanalysis. The reanalysis of the plan - as a whole, or in part - must be done whenever:

- there is a significant change made in the facility operations, which may create a new significant vulnerability
- there is new information about potential vulnerabilities associated with the food operation or facility;
- one or more mitigation strategies, or the food defense plan as a whole are not properly implemented;
- the FDA requires a reanalysis to respond to new vulnerabilities, credible threats and developments in the scientific understanding of food defense.

If none of the changes above happen, the frequency of the reanalysis must be at least once every 3 years.

Depending on the situation, the reanalysis must be done before any operational change is effective (including any change in mitigation strategies) or within 90 calendar days after production has started, or

If that timeframe cannot be respected, the food defense plan must include a written justification.

Record keeping

The food defense plan must be written in all its parts and include a description of all of the preparation and management activities, with several additional details such as:

- the training received by all the personnel in charge of applying the mitigation strategies or preparing the plan
- the entire vulnerability assessment, regardless of the outcome

- an explanation of why the chosen mitigation strategies will be effective
- a description of the monitoring procedures and their outcome, whether positive or negative
- the demonstration that mitigation strategies are working as intended
- justification of why the required timeframe for implementation could not be met.

The written description is considered part of the official records, and is subject to the same general requirements of the food safety plan (see chapter 6 for more details).

As a service to the reader we have created an Excel file containing all the hyperlinks which are mentioned in the book. You can download the Excel file via this link: https://www.foodsafety-experts.com/fsma-book-link/

Alternatively, you can also scan this QR code:

CHAPTER 9

Implementation Plan Intentional Adulteration and Food Defense

This chapter contains a table which you can use to plan the detailed steps to take towards compliance with the Intentional Adulteration Rule and Food Defence Rule.

The first column of the table identifies the company size, as not all actions are required for all types of companies. Please note that there is a difference in the definition of very small company in relation to Human Food and Animal Food: the first has a threshold of $1,000,000 average sales per year over the last 3 years, and the latter has a threshold of $2,5000,000 average sales per year over the last 3 years.

The second column provides the action to take towards compliance with these FSMA rules.

In the third column you can evaluate whether the action is relevant for your company, based on its size and the current status of FSMA compliance.

In the fourth column you can insert the action you are going to take, but before doing so – please read column five as well, as it contains valuable remarks in relation to the action to take.

In the last three columns you can assign actions to various people in your organization, includ-ing a deadline and a status update for regular review.

The table has been rotated by 90 degrees, so it maximizes the use of the paper and it allows you to make copies more easily. You can also download this table in an Excel file via this link: https://www.foodsafety-experts.com/fsma-book-excel/ . Alternatively, you can scan this QR-code:

Company Size	Item description	Relevant	Action	Remarks	Responsible	Due Date	Status
All	"Check whether your company is exempt from the Intential adulteration rule: - Holding of food, except holding of food in liquid storage tanks - Packing, re-packing, labeling, or re-labeling of food where the container that directly contacts the food remains intact - Produce Alcoholic beverages if such food: - Is in prepackaged form that prevents any direct human contact with such food - Constitutes not more than 5 percent of the overall sales of the facility, as determined by the Secretary of the Treasury"			If you are not exempt you need to perform the actions for small or large companies			
Large	Assess whether all individuals performing activities for the Intentional Adulteration Rule are qualified to do so			If necessary follow formal PCQI training (FSPCA approved)			
Large	Create and implement your Food Defense Policy and Procedures and records			See section 3 of chapter 8 for more details			
Large	Decide which tool to use (Food Defense Plan Builder, Carver+ Shock, SSAFE) or decide to create a VACPP manually			See section 3 of chapter 8 for more details			
Large	Implement training on intentional adulteration for employees working at actionable process steps and their supervisors			See section 3 of chapter 8 for more details			
Small	Implement the Intentional Adulteration Guideline as provided by the FDA			Use the Mitigation Strategies document of the FDA			
Very Small	"Check if you are exempt for the Intentional Adulteration Rule: - Is your company averaging less than $10.000.000 per year, in both sales of human food plus the market value of human food produced, processed, packed or held without sale (e.g. held for a fee)?"			You are only required to provide for official review, upon request, documentation sufficient to show that the facility qualifies for this exemption			

CHAPTER 10

Sanitary Transportation of Human and Animal Food

I. FSMA'S DEFINITION OF TRANSPORTATION

The provisions on Sanitary Transportation of Human and Animal Food are included subpart O of Chapter I of CFR 21.

At its most basic, transportation means moving animal or human food from one point to another inside US territory. FSMA, however, is only concerned with the movements of food that may affect its sanitary conditions. For example, food that is transported in a completely closed container is out of scope, unless it requires temperature control.

II. WHO IT APPLIES TO AND WHO IS EXEMPT

In general, Sanitary Transportations provisions apply to shippers, loaders, carriers and receivers who transport food inside the United States by motor or rail, whether or not the food is offered for, or enters interstate commerce.

- The four roles above are defined as follows:
- The shipper arranges transportation
- The loader loads the food onto the vehicle
- The carrier physically transports it (food delivery services, however, are exempt)
- The receiver receives it at any point in the United States, which may or may not be its destination

Of course, an individual may have more than one role. For example, the carrier may also be the loader and an importer of food who arranges its transportation within the US is also a shipper.

Specific exemptions apply to types of food, transportation activities or operators.

1.900 (b) (1) Food that is trans-shipped through the United States to another country.

1.900 (b) (2) Food that is imported for future export and is neither consumed nor distributed in the United States.

1.900 (b) (3) Meat, poultry and egg products, as they are regulated by other federal laws.

1.900 Cases where *transportation will not affect the sanitary conditions of food*, are excluded from the definition of 'transportation operations'. These are:

- Food completely enclosed in containers (however, if such food requires temperature control it *is* subject to the subpart)
- Compressed food gases (e.g. cylinders of carbon dioxide, nitrogen used in food and beverage products)
- Food contact substances
- Human food by-products to be used as animal food without further processing
- Live food animals except molluscan shellfish
- Any transportation activities performed by a farm

1.900 Shippers, loaders, receivers, or carriers with less than $500,000 of average annual revenue are considered non-covered businesses and therefore not subject to the subpart's provisions.

Additional Waivers

After the subpart on Sanitary Transportation was published, the FDA extended exemptions to other cases where existing regulations are already guaranteeing safe transportation procedures for human and animal food:

- Shippers, carriers and receivers holding valid permits under the NCIMS (National Conference on Interstate Milk Shipments) Grade A Milk Program, when transporting Grade A milk and products.
- Food establishments (e.g., retail stores, restaurants, and home grocery delivery, holding valid permits), when acting as receivers, shippers, or carriers delivering food to consumers.
- Molluscs and shellfish for entities holding valid state permits under the National Shellfish Sanitation Program.

III. SAFETY TRANSPORTATION REQUIREMENTS

There are both general and specific requirements for vehicles and transportation equipment, operations and individuals according to their roles.

General requirements

Vehicles and transportation equipment

- Their design, construction material and equipment must be suitable for the intended use
- They must be cleanable and maintained properly
- When not in operation, they must be stored in a way as to prevent contamination from pests or other hazards that may make food unsafe

Transportation operations

- They must ensure adequate temperature control and prevent cross-contamination with raw food, allergens or other non-food items.
- To create and maintain the right conditions, transporters may have to take measures such as hand-washing, segregation, isolation, or the use of packaging to protect food
- Adequate conditions and measures will depend on the type of food and its production stage
- The responsibility for compliance must be assigned to qualified supervisors

Transporters

- Whenever shippers, receivers, loaders, or carriers become aware that the food has become unsafe during transportation, they must take appropriate actions to ensure that it will not be distributed.

- When different operators work for the same company (e.g. when transportation is subcontracted to other carriers), they are free to adopt common, integrated, written procedures to make compliance and consistency easier

Specific requirements

Shippers

Food transportation is a micro-supply chain in itself, especially when different individuals perform the roles of shipper, carrier, loader and receiver. The first link of this chain is the shipper, who must implement several written procedures.

Before the shipment, such procedures must ensure that:

- vehicles and equipment used for transportation are in appropriate sanitary conditions
- the food is transported under adequate temperature control (i.e. use time-temperature loggers or use stickers on the outer packaging which will indicate temperature range violations and at a very minimum have a recording of the air temperature in the vehicle/ container itself).
- safety of transported food will not be compromised by a previous cargo

When such tasks, or part of them, are delegated to the carrier, it must be specified in a written agreement.

At the time of shipment, the shipper must notify in writing to the carrier and, when necessary, to the loader:

- the sanitary and design specifications of the vehicle and the equipment, including any cleaning procedures
- the operating temperature for temperature-sensitive food including, if necessary, the pre-cooling phase

A one-time notification is sufficient, unless procedures change, or a different type of food requires different procedures.

Loaders

Before loading food that is not completely enclosed by a container, the loader must determine that:

- the vehicle and transportation equipment are in appropriate sanitary and physical conditions and free of visible pest infestation
- the safety of transported food will not be compromised by a previous cargo
- the temperature control compartment works as intended and was properly pre-cooled, if necessary
- the vehicle and transportation equipment meet other sanitary conditions for food transportation

This assessment may be conducted by any appropriate means, following, if necessary, the specifications provided by the shipper.

Receivers

Upon receiving the food, receivers must verify that there was no significant temperature variation. They can do that by measuring the food's temperature, the ambient temperature of the vehicle and its temperature setting, or by conducting a sensory inspection.

Also, receivers have the right to ask carriers for specific information about the conditions of the food during transportation (see next section). C

Carriers

Carriers are responsible for the following tasks, whenever these are specified in a written agreement with the shipper:

- ensure that vehicles and transportation equipment meet the shipper's specifications
- once they reach their destination, provide the receiver, if requested, with the operating temperature specified by the shipper
- if requested by the receiver or the shipper, demonstrate that during transportation the food has maintained the temperature specified by the shipper
- pre-cool the cold storage compartment if the shipper requests it and following their specifications
- when they offer transportation with a bulk vehicle (which means that the food is directly in contact with the container) provide the shipper with information that identifies the previous cargo, and the most recent cleaning of the vehicle. The purpose is to prevent potential allergen cross-contamination and to preserve the kosher or halal status of the bulk vehicle

Additionally, a carrier must implement written procedures that:

- Specify sanitation and inspection practices of vehicles and equipment
- Describe how they will demonstrate that the temperature control was adequate during transportation, if requested by the receiver

Record keeping

All the written procedures, specifications and agreements mentioned in this chapter are considered part of the official records and subject to the general requirements (see chapter 4 for requirements details).

As a service to the reader we have created an Excel file containing all the hyperlinks which are mentioned in the book. You can download the Excel file via this link: https://www.foodsafety-experts.com/fsma-book-link/

Alternatively, you can also scan this QR code:

CHAPTER 11

Implementation Plan Sanitary Transport

This chapter contains a table which you can use to plan the detailed steps to take towards compliance with the Sanitary Transport Rule.

The first column of the table identifies the company size. You will notice that in this case the actions apply to all companies, irrespective of size.

The second column provides the action to take towards compliance with these FSMA rules.

In the third column you can evaluate whether the action is relevant for your company, based on the current status of FSMA compliance.

In the fourth column you can insert the action you are going to take, but before doing so – please read column five as well, as it contains valuable remarks in relation to the action to take.

In the last three columns you can assign actions to various people in your organization, includ-ing a deadline and a status update for regular review.

The table has been rotated by 90 degrees, so it maximizes the use of the paper and it allows you to make copies more easily. You can also download this table in an Excel file via this link: https://www.foodsafety-experts. com/fsma-book-excel/ . Alternatively, you can scan this QR-code:

Company Size	Item description	Relevant	Action	Remarks	Responsible	Due Date	Status
All	Create stakeholder management plan			Create a list of stakeholders and decide what actions you need to take involve the important stakeholders.			
All	Create the high level implementation plan			After reading the relevant chapters for your organization, you take all the relevant actions and combine these to a single plan. This way you will get a good indication of the overall timing of your implementation project.			
All	Create presentaton for senior management to gain buy in and approval						

Company Size	Item description	Relevant	Action	Remarks	Responsible	Due Date	Status
All	"Check whether you are exempt of the Sanitary Transport Rule: - Shippers, receivers, or carriers with transportation operations with less than $500,000 in average annual revenue - Transportation activities performed by a farm - Trans-shipments of food through the U.S. - Food not consumed in the U.S. (import for export) - Transportation of: - Food fully enclosed by a container (except if requiring temperature control) - Live food animals, except molluscan shellfish - Compressed food gases and food contact substances - Human food byproducts for use as animal food without further processing - Shippers, carriers and receivers holding valid permits under the NCIMS Grade A Milk Program, when transporting Grade A milk and products. - Food establishments, e.g., retail stores, restaurants, and home grocery delivery, holding valid permits, when acting as receivers, shippers, or carriers delivering food to consumers - Mollusks and shellfish for entities holding valid state permits under the National Shellfish Sanitation Program - Any additional waivers as published by the FDA "			If you are NOT exempt, please complete the actions below			
All	Verify whether all the detailed requirements are in place, using PowerPoint presentation of Module 5 - slides 28 to 31, including all downloads and links provided in the presentation						
All	Perform all required training activities as shown in the PowerPoint presentation of Module 5, slide 32						
All	Ensure all records are in place as shown in the PowerPoint presentation of Module 5, slide 33						

CHAPTER 12

The Produce Safety and Sprout Safety Rules

I. THE SPECIAL FOCUS ON E. COLI AND OTHER PATHOGENS

The purpose of the Produce Safety rule (full name: *Standards for The Growing, Harvesting, Packing, and Holding of Produce for Human Consumption*) is to provide specific requirements and practices to avoid contamination of produce. The rule covers all aspects of a farm's activity, such as hygiene and sanitising practices, the use of water, equipment and tools, wild and domesticated animals etc.

The Produce Safety rule is much more detailed compared to the one on Preventive Controls. While the HARPC process is somewhat flexible about the parameters and values that can be used as a reference for contaminations (provided these are based on scientific data), the Produce Safety rule indicates specific microbiological values and testing methods to follow. Three aspects of a farm's growing operations are particularly under scrutiny.

The safety of water and biological soil amendments of animal origin

The main focus here is on preventing contamination with E. coli, both in generic form and in the infamous O157:H7 variant. The bacteria are commonly found in animal faces - and water can be an efficient medium of transmission.

Contaminated produce is often the cause of serious E. coli outbreaks in the US. One of the latest examples at the time of writing is a multistate outbreak of E. coli O157:H7 linked to romaine lettuce, which infected at least 210 people in 36 states and caused 5 deaths.

The safety of sprouts

The rule includes additional provisions to avoid contamination of sprouts with E. coli, Listeria, Salmonella and other similarly dangerous pathogens.

The FDA explained the rationale for these additional requirements in the announcement of the draft guidance on sprouts operations:

Sprouts present a unique risk because the conditions under which they are typically produced are also ideal for the growth of bacteria that cause foodborne illnesses. Between 1996 and July 2016 there were 46 reported outbreaks associated with sprouts in the United States, accounting for 2474 illnesses, 187 hospitalizations, and three deaths.

II. HOW THE RULE IS ORGANISED

The rule is divided in 15 subparts going from A to R (G, H, and J are reserved). We included a short description of each below, following the order we presented them in this chapter, rather than the alphabetic order of the rule.

General Provisions (A) and General Requirements (B). They define general applicability and exclusions, and the overall purpose of the rule.

Personnel Qualifications and Training (C), Health and Hygiene (D), and Growing, Harvesting, Packing, and Holding Activities (K). Staff training is very important in FSMA and the Produce Safety rule is no exception. Subpart C provides the general training requirements, while the provisions on health and hygiene and growing operations in subparts D an K should also be considered a list of minimum topics a training should include.

Agricultural Water (E). This part includes provisions about safety standards for water and its distribution system. Standards may differ depending on the intended use.

Biological Soil Amendments of Animal Origin and Human Waste (F). In this subpart, special attention is dedicated to the prevention of E. coli contamination.

Domesticated and Wild Animals (I). Animals are not just a potential source of water contamination, they can also damage crops making them unsuitable for harvesting. This rule establishes what must be done to prevent contamination and specifies that wild animals should not be harmed or harassed to protect crops.

Equipment, Tools, Buildings, and Sanitation (L). This subpart covers the sanitation practices and the design requirements of equipment tools and buildings.

Sprouts (M). This subpart includes the additional requirements for growing sprouts. Also, we included some extra recommendations taken from the FDA's guidance.

Records (O). This subpart includes the general requirements regarding records and specific provisions that apply to farm operations.

Analytical Methods (N) and Variances (P). Subpart N provides details on what methods and standards farms must follow when conducting tests. The subpart is relatively short but highly technical, so it can be referenced to directly. Subpart P describes how and in what circumstances an independent entity (e.g. a state, tribe, or country) can be allowed to follow different standards.

Withdrawal of Qualified Exemption (R). The subpart describes the possible reasons for withdrawal of a qualified exemption and the withdrawal process.

Compliance and Enforcement (Q). This is a brief subpart with a few specifications about the definition of compliance and adulteration. We excluded it from the chapter as it does not contain any relevant information.

III. WHO IT APPLIES TO AND WHO IS EXEMPT

The rule's specific applications and exemptions depend on the type of produce and farms.

Covered and uncovered produce

In general, the rule applies to produce that is also a Raw Agricultural Commodity (RAC). 'Produce' means any fruit or vegetable and includes mushrooms, any type of sprouts, peanuts, tree nuts, and herbs. RAC is defined in section 201 of the Federal Food, Drug and Cosmetic Act as "any food in its raw or natural state." Produce RAC that is grown abroad and imported to the US is also subject to the rule.

At §112.1, the rule includes a detailed list of almost 100 types of covered fruits and vegetables.

Covered produce may be considered exempt if, after it is harvested, it is processed in a way that reduces microbiological hazards (for example, tomatoes used for producing tomato paste).

Such processing activities may be conducted by the same farm or by another entity further down the distribution chain. In that case, however, the farm must follow the customer written assurance process to qualify for the exemption (see chapter 4 for further details).

Uncovered produce is the one that:

- is grown for personal consumption
- is not a RAC
- is a RAC but is rarely consumed raw. The full list can be found at §112.2(a)(1).

What farms are covered

In general, the rule applies to all farms and farm mixed-type facilities, including packing houses (see chapter 2 for detailed definition of farms). However, small operations with less than $25,000 of average monetary value of sold produce are excluded. The average value is calculated on a rolling basis during the previous 3-year period and adjusted for inflation.

IV. REQUIREMENTS FOR TRAINING, HYGIENE, AND GROWING OPERATIONS

Training requirements

The basic principle about training is quite straightforward: everyone who handles produce or food contact surfaces must receive adequate training for their duties. This applies to employees and contractors, part-time, full-time and seasonal workers.

Personnel must be trained when they are hired, and then whenever appropriate, at least once a year after.

Depending on the tasks, three levels of training are required.

At the very minimum, everyone must receive training on:

- principles of food hygiene and food safety
- the importance of health and personal hygiene for staff and visitors
- recognizing symptoms of health conditions that may cause contamination

For harvesting staff, additional training is required on recognising possibly contaminated produce and inspecting harvest containers and equipment.

At least one of the supervisors must receive food safety training equivalent to a standard FDA curriculum.

Subparts D and K include provisions for staff health and hygiene and safety during growing operations but can also provide useful guidance on the minimum topics to include in training.

Hygiene requirements

Health and hygiene requirements focus on the three aspects.

People in charge of farming operations must exclude from work personnel with any health condition that may cause contamination, like infection, open lesion, vomiting, or diarrhoea) and instruct workers to report any possibility of being ill.

Personnel must keep adequate personal cleanliness, take appropriate measures in case of direct contact with working animals and avoid contact with all other animals. A lot of details are provided about hand-washing procedures and the use of gloves.

Farm staff must inform visitors of health and hygiene procedures and make sure they follow them. Also, visitors must have access to toilets and hand-washing facilities.

Growing operations requirements

Growing operations include growing, harvesting, packing and holding.

- Farms that grow, harvest, pack or hold both covered and uncovered produce must keep the two separated until the moment they are distributed. Also, food contact surfaces that are used for both types of produce must be kept clean at all times.

- Harvesting staff must identify produce that is likely to be contaminated and not harvest it. At a minimum, the assessment must be about possible or actual contamination of animal excrement and requires a visual inspection, regardless of the harvesting method.
- Produce that drops to the ground before harvest must not be distributed. This of course excludes roots, root crops or crops that must be dropped to the ground to be harvested, like almonds and olives.
- Harvested produce must be handled in such a way to avoid possible contamination.
- During packaging operations, farms must pay particular attention to the possible formation of Clostridium Botulinum toxin (if that is a foreseeable hazard).
- Food packing and packaging materials must be food-grade, designed for single use or, if reusable, cleanable and cleaned before each use.

V. AGRICULTURAL WATER

In general, water used in farms must be safe for the intended use. The rule provides specific provisions and standards to avoid E. coli contamination. Such standards vary depending on the intended use.

Maintenance of sources, distribution systems, and pooling of water

For the part of the water distribution system under their control (including facilities and equipment), farms must conduct an inspection at least once a year at the beginning of the growing season and do regular maintenance throughout the year.

Inspections must focus on:

- the nature of each water source
- the extent of farm's control over them
- their degree of protection
- how adjacent and nearby land is used
- the likelihood of introduction of hazards by another user before water reaches the farm

Safety standards for agricultural water

The rule is flexible about what water treatment method farms should follow, provided it is consistently effective and its efficacy is regularly monitored.

The standard of reference indicated by the FDA is the EPA Method 1603. The rule provides specific microbiological values based on 100ml of samples.

No detectable presence of generic E. coli is allowed when water is:

- used for irrigating sprouts
- applied to produce during or after harvesting
- applied to food contact surfaces
- used for washing hands

When water is used for irrigating produce (excluding sprouts), the maximum tolerated values of E. coli are:

- A geometric mean (GM) of 126 colony-forming units (CFU)
- A statistical threshold value (STV) of 410 CFU (STV basically measures how values change over time)

Sprouts are excluded from these tolerance levels because they are harvested very close to the soil - sometimes even including the soil –, therefore the risk of E. coli migration onto the product is higher. This is further enhanced by the fact that sprouts are mostly consumed raw.

When E. coli is detected in water intended for uses where no presence of the bacteria is tolerated, farms must immediately stop using it.

After that, they can choose if either treat the water or reinspect the entire distribution system, identify the source of contamination, take necessary measures and verify their effectiveness.

If water used for irrigating produce has a presence of E. coli values above the limits, farms must stop using it as soon as practicable, but at the latest within one year. To avoid that, they can choose one of these three options:

a) To use time intervals to allow the bacteria to die off on the field. The interval can be between the last irrigation and harvest (but for no more than four consecutive days) or between harvest and the end of storage. Additionally, farms can use other activities (such as washing) to make sure microbiological levels return below the threshold. At §112.45 the rule specifies what die-off rate criteria to follow.

b) Reinspect the entire water distribution system, take necessary measures and verify that they were effective.
c) Treat the water.

When and how often farms must test water

When water was treated to eliminate any detectable trace of E. coli, farms are exempt from testing it.

Water is considered pre-treated when it is sanitised directly by farms (using methods considered adequate) or comes from a public water system. In the latter case, however, farms must provide certificates of compliance or results from the provider proving that the water has no detectable trace of E. coli.

When water is untreated, testing requirements depend on the intended use. All samples must be collected aseptically.

For uses where no detectable presence of E. coli is allowed, farms must initially test each source at least four times during the growing season or over a period of one year, using at least 4 samples in each test. If they return no presence of E. coli, farms can repeat them once a year, this time with a minimum of one sample. If tests fail, they must start from scratch with an initial test.

Untreated water used for irrigating produce (other than sprouts) follows a slightly different procedure. An important difference is between surface water (the one found in lakes, rivers and streams) and ground water (whose source is located underground).

Testing surface water. For the initial survey, farms will collect a minimum of twenty samples in a period between two and four years. These samples will be used to calculate the GM and STV. For the annual survey there must be a minimum of five samples. Together with the fifteen most recent samples, these will form a rolling data set to be used to update GM and STV values.

Testing ground water. For the initial survey, farms will collect a minimum of four samples as close as practicable to harvest, during the growing season or over a period of one year. These samples will be used to calculate the GM and STV. For the annual survey, they will collect a minimum of one sample. Together with the three most recent samples, these will form a rolling data set to be used to update GM and STV values.

Can farms use alternative criteria?

Farms are allowed to use alternative criteria to determine microbial quality, microbial die-off rate and time interval, and the minimum number of samples for the initial and annual survey of untreated surface water. However, they must show scientific data proving that the alternative methods would provide the same level of public health protection as those indicated by the FDA.

VI. BIOLOGICAL SOIL AMENDMENTS

Biological soil amendments are biological agents added the soil to improve plant development and can derive from plants, animals or humans. The Produce Safety rule includes no limitations to the use of plant-based amendments, only allows treated human waste (sewage sludge), and strictly regulates the use of soil amendments of animal origin in subpart F.

This subpart focuses on three aspects: treatment, storing and application.

Treatment of soil amendments of animal origin

A soil amendment of animal origin is considered treated when it goes through a process that eliminates any presence of Listeria, Salmonella and E. coli O157:H7 according to specific testing criteria specified at §112.55.

The rule provides two sets of standards: one considers all three bacteria (no presence allowed) while the other only considers Salmonella (no presence allowed) and a specific tolerance for the presence of faecal coliforms. Compliance with one or the other will then determine the procedure to follow to apply the amendment to the soil.

As an additional requirement, when the soil amendment is agricultural tea (which is a water extract of biological materials), the brewing water cannot have any detectable presence of E. coli and the tea cannot be brewed using untreated surface water.

A soil amendment of animal origin is considered untreated if:

- it did not go through treatment process
- it became contaminated after treatment or there is good reason to believe it did
- after treatment it was mixed with untreated amendments of animal origin

165

- it contains untreated waste that could pose a health hazard
- it is agricultural tea that contains an additive

Application of soil amendments of animal origin

The procedure to apply soil amendments changes slightly depending on whether it is treated or not and, if treated, what set of standards it complies with.

- If it is untreated, application must avoid any contact with covered produce during or after application
- If it complies with the standards for Salmonella and specific coliforms, application must minimise contact with produce.
- If it complies with *standards for Listeria, Salmonella and E. coli O157:H7,* no restrictions apply.

Storing of biological soil amendments

Any biological soil amendment of animal origin (whether treated or untreated) must be stored in a way not to contaminate produce, food contact surfaces, areas, water sources or distribution systems, and other soil amendments. Also, storage must minimise the risk of contamination by untreated or in-process biological soil amendment of animal origin.

VII. WILD AND DOMESTICATED ANIMALS

Subpart I applies to those situations where produce is grown outdoor or in a partially-enclosed building and there is a reasonable probability that domesticated or wild animals contaminate the produce.

Produce grown in greenhouses or other fully enclosed buildings is excluded, as well as fish used in aquaculture operations.

Farms in this case are required to control if any produce could have been contaminated or destroyed by any animal. If there is reason to believe it happened, harvesting personnel must avoid harvesting produce that is unsuitable.

To avoid any possible misinterpretation, the subpart specifies that under no circumstances farms are required to kill, harm or pursue endangered species, or take measures to keep animals away from the fields.

VIII. EQUIPMENT, TOOLS AND BUILDINGS

General requirements

This subpart applies to any tool or piece of equipment that has any form of contact with produce during a farming activity. That can be anything from knives to mechanical harvesters. Buildings are any structure, fully or partially enclosed, with wall or not, that is used for farming activities or to store food contact surfaces.

Equipment and tools must be designed and manufactured in a way to be cleanable. Their seams must minimise accumulation of dirt and other potential contaminants. Also, they must be maintained properly and inspected regularly, cleaned and sanitised whenever necessary.

Non-food contact surfaces must be kept clean during harvesting and other post-harvest activities.

Specific requirements

Instruments and controls must be accurate and precise, adequately maintained and used in adequate number for the designated use.

Transportation equipment must be adequately cleaned before use in transporting produce and adequate for the intended use.

Buildings must be suitable in size, construction and design to facilitate maintenance and sanitary operations and reduce the potential for contamination.

Their design must allow to keep potentially hazardous operations separated, by allowing them to take place in different locations or times, within enclosed systems, or by other effective means. In general, their design must allow to take proper precautions to reduce the potential for contamination.

In general, floors, walls, ceilings, fixtures, ducts, or pipes must be designed and maintained in a way to prevent contamination, including from dripping or condensation.

They must ensure adequate drainage in all areas where there is normal discharge of water or other liquid waste.

They must provide enough space for placement of equipment and storage of materials;

Farms must take all reasonable precautions to block *access of domesticated animals to fully-enclosed buildings.* Fully-enclosed building used for animals must be kept separated from farming areas.

Guard or guide dogs may be allowed if their presence is unlikely to result in contamination of produce, food contact surfaces, or food-packing materials.

To avoid *pest* contamination, farms must take necessary measures to exclude pests from fully-enclosed buildings and prevent them from becoming established.

Toilet facilities must be readily accessible to personnel, including around growing areas during harvesting activities.

They must be designed, located, and maintained in a way to:

- prevent contamination with human waste of covered produce, food contact surfaces, farming areas, water sources
- be serviced and cleaned with adequate frequency, and supplied with toilet paper
- allow for a safe waste disposal (waste water and toilet paper)

Hand-washing facilities must be located near toilet facilities during any farming activity that takes place in a fully-enclosed building. They must be furnished with:

- Soap or other effective surfactant, except antiseptic hand rubs
- Running water that satisfies the sanitary requirements (no detectable presence of *E. coli*)
- Adequate drying devices

Also, they must allow for the safe disposal of waste water and towels.

Regarding sewage, trash, litter, and waste (including of domesticated animals), farms are required to:

- Handle and dispose of them into adequate systems or through other adequate means
- Maintain such systems in a way that prevents contamination
- Manage dispose of leakages or spills of human waste in a manner that prevents contamination
- Ensure that such systems continue to operate as intended after a significant event (such as flooding or an earthquake) that could damage them

Plumbing must:

- Be of an adequate size and design
- Be adequately installed and maintained
- Distribute water under pressure as needed, where needed and in sufficient quantities
- Properly convey sewage and liquid disposable waste
- Avoid being a source of contamination
- Avoid backflow or cross connections that may cause contamination of agricultural water with waste water.

IX. SPROUTS

General and specific requirements

The subpart applies to all activities associated to sprouts (growing, harvesting, packing, and holding), including the seeds or beans used to grow them. The rule does not apply to substrate-grown sprouts harvested without their roots, like Alfalfa, soy bean sprouts, mung bean sprouts.

The general requirements for farms regarding sprouts are:

- To conduct all growing activities (growing, harvesting, packing and holding) in fully-enclosed buildings
- To clean and sanitise any food contact surface before contact with sprouts, seeds or beans used to grow them
- To visually inspect each lot of seeds and beans received from suppliers (included the packaging), for signs of potential contamination

The subpart includes specific provisions for:

- Treatment of seeds and beans
- Maintaining a written monitoring plan
- Testing sprouts for the presence of pathogens
- Taking specific actions if tests are positive

Treatment of seeds and beans

Treatment of seeds and beans used for sprouts is mandatory and must be conducted with a scientifically valid method that eliminates the risk of presence of pathogens. It can be done directly by farms or by their suppliers. In the latter case, farms must receive documentation from suppliers about the type of treatment and how seeds and beans were handled after the treatment.

Whenever there is reason to believe that a lot of seeds or beans was contaminated, farms must stop using them immediately and report the incident (and all findings) to the supplier.

Discontinuing seeds or beans is not necessary if these will be treated. However, the findings must still be reported to the supplier. Neither action is necessary if during further investigations, it is discovered that the lot was not in fact the source of contamination.

Testing

Farms must conduct two types of testing activities. In both cases samples must be collected aseptically.

Environmental testing during all growing activities for the presence of Listeria species or L. monocytogenes.

If tests are positive, the minimum corrective actions farms must take are:

- Conduct additional testing of surfaces and areas surrounding the area
- Clean and sanitize the affected surfaces and surrounding areas
- Conduct additional sampling
- Conduct finished product testing when appropriate
- Take any other necessary action to prevent the contamination from happening again
- Ensure that the sprouts are not distributed to the public

Test spent sprout irrigation water from each production batch for E. coli O157:H7, Salmonella species, plus any pathogens that could cause adverse health consequences. If testing spent water is not practicable (for example when sprouts are grown in soil or hydroponically with very little water), it must be conducted during production.

If tests are positive, the minimum corrective actions farms must take are:

- Follow the treatment procedure for seeds or beans used to grow the contaminated batch
- Clean and sanitise the affected surfaces and surrounding areas
- Take any other necessary action to prevent the contamination from happening again
- Ensure that the sprouts are not distributed to the public.

The environmental monitoring and sampling plans

Farms are required to maintain two written plans with all details of their monitoring and testing activities.

An environmental monitoring plan for the detection of Listeria species or L. monocytogenes. The plan must include details about:

- What pathogens the test is for
- How often environmental samples will be collected (which must be at least once a month) and at what production stage.
- Where samples will be collected. Sampling must be in adequate quantity and include food and non-food contact surfaces present in the environment where sprouts are growing.
- What corrective actions will be taken

A sampling plan for the detection of E. coli, Salmonella and other applicable pathogens in spent irrigation water. The plan must include details about the number and location of samples for each production batch and corrective actions to take.

Further details on how to implement sprout requirements

After publishing the Produce Safety rule, the FDA also provided a guidance on the implementation of sprout requirements, which contains specific recommendations for each phase of the sprout production process. Below, we included a few important recommendations taken from the guidance.

Cleaning & sanitizing of food contact surfaces. Cleaning and sanitising are two distinct steps. Cleaning is about removing visible organic material and other debris from a surface, while sanitising means treating it in a way to destroy vegetative cells of undesirable microorganisms without making food unsafe. A surface must be clean before it can be sanitised.

Cleaning and sanitising food contact surfaces is required before any contact with sprouts, seeds or beans and is also part of the minimum corrective actions to take if tests reveal a contamination with hazardous pathogens. The minimum frequency recommended by the FDA is at least once a day (even when the food contact surface was not used for more than a day), or between each production batch.

The FDA also recommends conducting verification sampling of recently cleaned and sanitized surfaces to monitor the overall effectiveness of sanitation.

Seed Receiving, Handling and Storage. Seeds for sprouting should be grown under GAP (Good Agricultural Practices), although this is not a requirement of the rule. The FDA recommends conducting the visual examination upon

receipt and immediately reject them and contact the supplier if there is any sign of damage or contamination.

Environmental monitoring plan. Other than the minimum requirements, farms are recommended to add further details regarding:

- Test Methods used
- The person(s) responsible for sample collection and any specific training they should have
- Sample collection method and sample sizes to be collected
- The laboratory that conducts testing
- The records to be kept

Sampling and testing plan. Other than the minimum requirements, farms are recommended to add further details regarding:

- What pathogens the test is for
- Water used for irrigation such irrigation flow rates and number of drainage points.
- Whether testing is for SSIW (sprout spent irrigation water) or in-process sprouts and volume per each sample
- Volume of SSIW or quantity of sprouts used for testing. The recommended quantity is 1.5 litres or 1500 grams respectively
- Testing Methods used
- Timing of sample collection

X ANALYTICAL METHODS AND VARIANCES

Analytical methods

Subpart N includes technical details about what scientific methods should be used during the following activities:

- Testing agricultural water
- Environmental monitoring for sprouts
- Testing spent irrigation water for sprouts

Farms can use alternative methods to those indicated, provided that their efficacy is at least equivalent.

VARIANCES

A state, tribe, or country can request variances to the requirements of the rule, if it concludes that meeting one or more of the rule's requirements would be problematic, considering its local growing conditions.

In this case, a person or organization that is the regulatory authority for that entity must submit a request of variance through a petition where it demonstrates that the requested variance is reasonably likely to ensure that the produce is not adulterated and provides the same level of public health protection as the corresponding requirement(s) in the rule.

XI. QUALIFIED EXEMPTIONS ELIGIBILITY AND REASONS FOR WITHDRAWAL

The Produce Safety rule also allows certain small and very small businesses to follow simplified requirements with a qualified exemption.

To be considered a small or very small farm, the average monetary value of food sold in the previous 3-year must be up to $500,000, calculated as rolling average and adjusted for inflation. Additionally, to receive a qualified exemption most of the food must be sold to qualified end-users, as opposed to other businesses (see chapter 4 for further details).

Other than subpart R on withdrawal of qualified exemption, entitled farms are only subject to:

- General Provisions
- Subpart O on records
- Subpart Q on compliance and enforcement
- Subpart R on withdrawal of qualified exemption

They are exempt from all the rest of the subparts. However, they are subject to additional requirements whenever they sell or distribute food that would otherwise be covered by the rule.

When a food packaging label *is required*, it must show the name and the complete business address of the farm.

When a food packaging label *is not required* farms must display, at the point of purchase and at the moment of delivery, their name and complete business address on a label, poster, sign, placard, documents or in an electronic notice in the case of Internet sales.

In either case, this display of information must be "prominent and conspicuous."

All the supporting information that was provided to be granted the exemption must be kept for as long as necessary. The general 2-year retention period will not apply in this case.

Reasons for withdrawal

The FDA may issue a withdrawal in the event of an active investigation of a foodborne illness outbreak that is directly linked to the farm, or simply "based on conduct or conditions associated" with the farm, if such action is necessary to protect public health.

Although the withdrawal is the most drastic measure, the FDA may decide to take other actions, like a warning letter, a recall etc., also considering what corrective actions that were taken by the farm.

The withdrawal process follows a specific procedure, which is detailed in the subpart. Farms that were subject to withdrawal can appeal the FDA's decision.

XII. RECORDS

General requirements

Most of the general requirements for records are the same as those we have seen in the Preventive Controls rule.

All documentation must be created at the time an activity is performed, be accurate, legible, indelible, in true copies and include:

- Farm name and location
- The date and time of the documented activity
- The location of the growing area where the activity is taking place, whether it is a field, a building or a shed
- An adequate description of the produce the activity is related to (e.g. commodity name, brand name or lot number.

- The actual values and observations obtained during monitoring

Additionally, the supporting documentation for the following parts must be reviewed, dated, and signed by a qualified individual within a reasonable time frame:

- qualified exemption
- training
- inspections tests, treatments of agricultural water and time intervals or other actions to reduce presence of E. coli
- treatment of biological soil amendments of animal origin
- cleaning and sanitizing of equipment
- treatment of seeds and beans used for sprouts, as well as all analytical tests and corrective actions taken

Specific documentation to be included in records

In addition to the general requirements, most of the subparts we have described so far have a specific set of documents to be included.

Training: topics covered, and the persons(s) trained.

Agricultural water:

- The findings of the inspections of the water system
- Results of all analytical tests
- Results of water treatment
- Supporting scientific data or information for methods used for testing, treatment, time interval, or other activities used to reduce the presence of E. coli

- Details about the application of time interval or (calculated) log reduction, e.g. how it was determined and the dates of corresponding activities (last irrigation, harvest, end of storage, or commercial washing)
- Certificates of compliance from a public water system

Treated biological soil amendments of animal origin. When the soil amendment comes from a supplier, the documentation must be renewed at least annually and certify that:

- The process is scientifically valid and that appropriately monitored
- The soil amendment has been handled, conveyed and stored in such a way to minimise the risk of contamination by an untreated or in-process biological soil amendment of animal origin

When the soil amendment is produced by the farm, the documentation must prove that process controls (for example, time, temperature, and turnings) were achieved.

Equipment tools buildings and sanitation. Details about the date and methods used for cleaning and sanitising of equipment used for growing operations for sprouts and harvesting, packing, or holding activities.

Sprouts:

- Details about the type of treatment applied to seeds or beans. When treatment is applied by a supplier, the documentation must also confirm that seeds and beans were appropriately handled and packaged after the treatment

- The environmental monitoring plan
- The sampling plan
- The results of all analytical compliance tests
- Scientific supporting data about any alternative analytical methods used
- Details about any corrective actions that were taken
- Date and method used for cleaning and sanitising

How and for how long to keep records

- Records can be kept offsite, provided they can be retrieved in 24 hours
- If the farm is already keeping documentation with the relevant information in compliance with other local of federal regulations, there will not be any need to duplicate it
- If new information is added that complements the one in existing documentation, it can be included in a different set of records
- Records must be kept for two years, even when they are related to discontinued equipment or processes
- Documentation that supports qualified exemption, must be retained for as long as necessary

As a service to the reader we have created an Excel file containing all the hyperlinks which are mentioned in the book. You can download the Excel file via this link: https://www.foodsafety-experts.com/fsma-book-link/

Alternatively, you can also scan this QR code:

CHAPTER 13

Implementation Plan Produce Safety and Sprout Safety

T his chapter contains a table which you can use to plan the detailed steps to take towards compliance with the Produce Safety Rule and the Sprout Safety Rule.

The first table on the next three pages in this chapter combines the actions in relation to the Produce Safety Rule. The second table on the last two pages of this chapter contains all the actions in relation to the Sprout Safety Rule.

The first column of the table identifies the company size (all, small or very small), as not all actions are required for all types of companies.

The second column provides the action to take towards compliance with these FSMA rules.

In the third column you can evaluate whether the action is relevant for your company, based on its size and the current status of FSMA compliance.

In the fourth column you can insert the action you are going to take, but before doing so – please read column five as well, as it contains valuable remarks in relation to the action to take.

In the last three columns you can assign actions to various people in your organization, includ-ing a deadline and a status update for regular review.

The table has been rotated by 90 degrees, so it maximizes the use of the paper and it allows you to make copies more easily. You can also download this table in an Excel file via this link: https://www.foodsafety-experts. com/fsma-book-excel/ . Alternatively, you can scan this QR-code:

Company Size	Item description	Relevant	Action	Remarks	Responsible	Due Date	Status
All	Create stakeholder management plan			Create a list of stakeholders and decide what actions you need to take involve the important stakeholders.			
All	Create the high level implementation plan			After reading the relevant chapters for your organization, take all the relevant actionlists and combine these to a single plan. This way you will get a good indication of the overall timing of your implementation project.			
All	Create presentaton for senior management to gain buy in and approval						
All	All farm related activities under the scope of the Sprout Safety Rule are exempt from the Intentional Adulteration Rule						
All	Perform supplier risk assessment and determine supplier verification activities			See section 2 of chapter 6 for more details			
All	Determine whether your qualified individual needs formal, FDA approved training or document that the person is qualified based on experience, training and education received in the past.						

185

Company Size	Item description	Relevant	Action	Remarks	Responsible	Due Date	Status
All	"Check whether you are exempt for the Spout Safety Rule: - The Sprout Safety Rule applies to growing, harvesting, packing and holding of all sprout types except sprouts harvested above the soil or substrate line without their roots - Sprouts sold with roots attached, e.g., wheatgrass in a tray, are subject to subpart M, however, if sold to a customer who will harvest without roots, you can be exempt PROVIDED you annually collect written assurances from the customer"			If you are NOT exempt you need to complete all the actions below			
All	Review and adjust your cleaning and sanitization processes and procedures			See section 9 of chapter 12 for more details			
All	Review and adjust your seed receipt and treatment processes and procedures			See section 9 of chapter 12 for more details			
All	Review your water sampling & testing and environmental monitoring processes and procedures			See section 9 of chapter 12 for more details			
All	Ensure all records are in place in relation to the Sprout Safety Rule			See section 12 of chapter 12 for more details			
All	Conduct the required training for all staff			See section 4 of chapter 12 for more details			

CHAPTER 14

Training for FSMA Compliance

I. GENERAL PRINCIPLES OF TRAINING

In FSMA, any individual involved in the food supply chain must be qualified to perform their assigned duties. This requirement applies to employees and contractors, permanent and seasonal workers.

Depending on the circumstances, an individual's qualification may be based mainly on education, work experience, or training, or a mix of the three. Here are a few specific examples.

Education:

- Degree in Food Safety, Food Processing
- Specific university courses (e.g., on microbiology or food allergens)

Work experience:

- 5 or more years in the same line of industry
- More than 3 years in a GFSI-certified site
- 5 or more years of auditing experience (e.g. 3rd party auditing or supplier auditing), preferably with specific training

Training:

- FDA-approved training
- Other training combinations:
  - The FSMA Masterclass related to this book
  - Relevant HACCP training
  - Food Microbiology relevant to the products and ingredients
  - Allergens Management Training
  - Self-study of FDA-approved training material

II. SPECIFIC TRAINING REQUIREMENTS

Preventive Controls, FSVP and VQIP

For the rules on Preventive Controls on human and animal food and the supply chain programs for domestic and foreign suppliers, FSMA includes a staged training model.

Qualified Individuals and supervisors

All individuals who manufacture, process, pack, or hold food must receive training in the principles of food hygiene and food safety. This includes the importance of employee health and personal hygiene, as appropriate to the food, the facility and the individual's assigned duties.

Additionally, facilities must provide specific training to those employees working at process steps with preventive controls. Whenever there is an existing HACCP program in place, they can simply extend training on CCPs to the rest of preventive controls.

Supervisory personnel must have the necessary qualification to ensure the application of food hygiene and safety practices.

Preventive Controls Qualified Individual (PCQI)

The task of PCQIs is to prepare and implement all parts of the food safety plan or to oversee such activities. Because of the importance of their role, they are required to have a higher level of qualification.

A Preventive Controls Qualified Individual must have successfully completed training in the development and application of risk-based preventive controls. The training can be a standard FDA curriculum, or one equivalent. Alternatively, qualification can also come through relevant job experience.

Qualified Auditor

Following the same principle as the Qualified Individual, a quality auditor must have the relevant technical expertise to be able to perform the audit either by training or have acquired the necessary technical expertise through education, training, experience, or a combination thereof.

Dealing with foreign suppliers

Individuals in charge of the Foreign Supplier Verification Program or the Voluntary Qualified Importer Program must also be able to read and understand the language of any records coming from foreign suppliers.

Intentional Adulteration and Food Defence

For the rule on Mitigation Strategies against Intentional Adulteration, FSMA has a similar training model as for the preventive controls.

Qualified Individuals and supervisors

Individuals assigned to actionable process steps must have adequate qualification and receive training in food defence awareness.

Supervisory personnel must have the necessary qualification to ensure the application of mitigation strategies.

Food defence team

Individuals in charge of preparing and implementing the food defence plan (or overseeing such activities) must be qualified individuals who have successfully completed training for their function. Such training can be based on the standard, FDA-approved, curriculum or an equivalent one and includes relevant work experience.

Transport safety

In the Sanitary Transportation rule, carriers must be provided with adequate and documented training on sanitary transportation practices and awareness of potential food safety problems that may occur during food transportation. In practical terms, it means that loaders, truck drivers and receivers must be trained in sanitary transportation practices and on how to prevent and detect food safety issues.

Produce Safety rule

Basic training

All personnel must receive adequate training depending on their duties, including:

- principles of food hygiene and food safety
- the importance of health and personal hygiene, including recognising symptoms of health conditions that could result in contamination
- the relevant standards under the Produce Safety rule that are applicable to the employee's job responsibilities

Harvesting staff

Personnel in charge of harvesting produce must receive additional training on:

- recognizing produce that must not be harvested, including covered produce that may be contaminated
- inspecting harvest containers and equipment to ensure that they are functioning properly, clean, and maintained so as not to become a source of contamination
- correcting problems with harvest containers or equipment, or reporting such problems to the supervisor (or other responsible party), as appropriate to the person's job responsibilities

Supervisors

Although there is no Qualified Individual in the Produce Safety rule, at least one supervisor must have successfully completed food safety training equivalent to the standardised Produce Safety Alliance curriculum.

III. THE FDA TRAINING NETWORK

In order to fulfil all the training requirements around the globe, the FDA has engaged with 3 alliances to create, deliver and maintain the relevant training materials.

Next to these alliances, there are cooperative agreements with institutions in the USA to deliver knowledge and training to farmers as these are the biggest group.

Finally, the FDA set up three regional coordination centres in the USA for general support around FSMA, as well as a collaboration with the International Food Protection Training Institute for training support outside the USA.

Alliances

- Food Safety Preventive Controls Alliance (FSPCA)
- Produce Safety Alliance (PSA)
- Sprout Safety Alliance (SSA)

Cooperative agreements

- National Farmers Union Foundation
- University of Arkansas at Fayetteville
- National Association of State Departments of Agriculture (NASDA)

Coordination Centres

- University of Florida (south)
- Oregon State University (west)
- Iowa State University (north central)
- University of Vermont and State Agricultural College (north east)

IV. TRAINING RESOURCES

Although certified training is not a legal requirement in FSMA, it can be a valid solution for individuals without the necessary education or experience.

Training resources on preventive controls

The FSPCA offers three different types of training for preventive controls on human and animal food:

- Live PCQI training (2-3 days in a classroom)
- Blended PCQI training (delivered online with one day in a classroom)
- Lead Instructor training. The requirements to have access to this training are:
  - To have successfully completed the PCHF/PCAF training
  - To be an approved FSPCA Lead Instructor candidate. Registration must be submitted through this link: https://fspca.force.com/FSPCA/s/li-public-guidance?language=en_US

The FSPCA provides a database with a list of accredited agencies and the details of the type of training they provide: https://fspca.force.com/FSPCA/s/courselist?language=en_US

Training resources on food defence

For food defence, the essentials are included in the PCHF and PCAF training and there are a few additional training courses provided by the FDA:

FSPCA Food Defense Awareness for the IA Rule

https://www.ifsh.iit.edu/sites/ifsh/files/departments/
fspca/pdfs/FSPCA_IA_FoodDefenseAwareness_
Information-Sheet_05-29-18.pdf

FSPCA Overview of the Intentional Adulteration Rule

https://www.ifsh.iit.edu/sites/ifsh/files/departments/
fspca/pdfs/FSPCA_IA_Rule_Overview_Information-
Sheet_06-26-18.pdf

Training resources on produce safety

The Produce Safety Alliance Grower Training Course has approximately seven hours of educational material divided in the following seven modules:

- Introduction to Produce Safety
- Worker Health, Hygiene, and Training
- Soil Amendments
- Wildlife, Domesticated Animals, and Land Use
- Agricultural Water (Part I: Production Water; Part II: Postharvest Water)
- Postharvest Handling and Sanitation
- How to Develop a Farm Food Safety Plan

This training is available both in the US and internationally. For individuals based in the US, this link provides an overview of upcoming training courses: https://producesafetyalliance.cornell.edu/training/grower-training-courses/upcoming-grower-trainings

The list of certified trainers outside the US can be consulted at this page: https://fm71.triple8.net/fmi/webd/#Trainer-Directory

Training on produce safety also has two more tiers.

Training course to become a trainer: https://producesafetyalliance.cornell.edu/training/train-trainer-course/psa-trainer-and-lead-trainer-process

Training course to become a trainer of trainers: https://producesafetyalliance.cornell.edu/training/train-trainer-course/tots

JIFSAN portal.

Next to the Sprout Safety Alliance Training, the FDA teamed up with the university of Maryland and created the JIFSAN Training Portal on food defence, with specific training on:

- Aquaculture Drugs and US Regulations Training Module for International Producers
- Develop Your Food Protection Plan
- Hazard Analysis and Critical Control Point
- Pesticide Module: Validation and Verification
- Pesticide Residue Analysis: Mass Spectrometry
- Pesticide Residue Analysis: Sample Preparation and Chromatography
- Pesticide Residue Analysis: Tolerances and Compliance
- Food Safety Training for Farm Workers: Spices and Dried Aromatic Herbs

Training resources on sprout safety

The Sprout Safety Association created a Sprouter Training Course in live format (two days in a classroom) or blended format (8-12 hours on-line, plus one day of live training).

There is also a Lead Instructor course available, also in either live or blended format.

To access this training, individuals must prove to have basic knowledge and experience in one or more of the following areas:

- Biological sciences; food science /technology; microbiology
- Work experience in food safety
- Knowledge of sprouting operations and understand sprout production and food safety risks that could exist in sprout production environment
- Knowledge of the FSMA Produce Safety Rule
- Teaching experience in adult learning

This page provides all relevant information: https://www.ifsh.iit.edu/ssa/resources/ssa-training

As a service to the reader we have created an Excel file containing all the hyperlinks which are mentioned in the book. You can download the Excel file via this link: https://www.foodsafety-experts.com/fsma-book-link/

Alternatively, you can also scan this QR code:

About The Authors

ROB KOOIJMANS

Rob Kooijmans has over 22 years of experience in the international food industry and he has held various senior positions as QA director and VP QA. He has worked for large multi-nationals like Unilever and DSM and also for large privately held companies like Farm Frites. For over 4 years Rob is the co-founder and co-owner of FoodRecall.nl - a boutique consulting agency 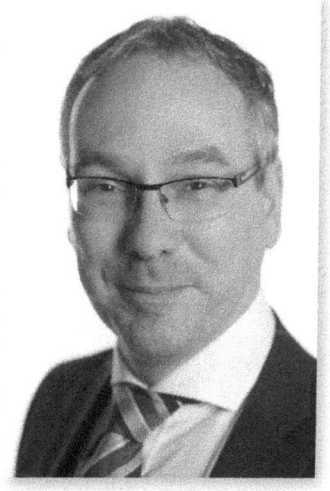 for the food sector and Food Safety Experts - an on-line training and coaching business aimed at quality managers in the international food industry. Rob is a celebrated speaker and author in the areas of quality and food safety.

KITTY APPELS

Kitty Appels has over 25 years of experience in the international food industry and she has a wealth of international experience with a vast range of companies, among which Friesland Campina, Heineken, Merieux Nutrisciences, Ausnutria, ADM and Henkel. For over 4 years Kitty is the 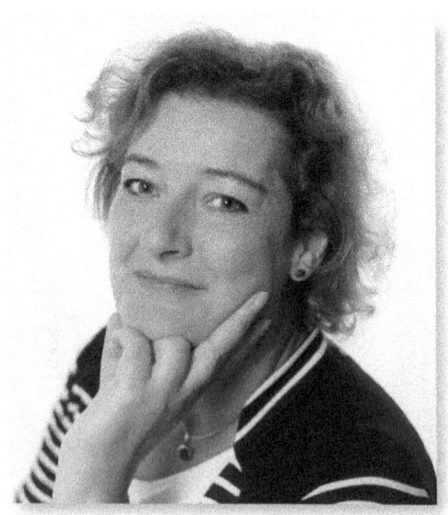 co-founder and co-owner of FoodRecall.nl - a boutique consulting agency for the food sector and Food Safety Experts - an on-line training and coaching business aimed at quality managers in the international food industry. Kitty is an international speaker and author in the areas of quality and food safety.

FOOD SAFETY EXPERTS – WHAT WE STAND FOR

You as owner of a food company or a as quality or food safety professional are filled with PASSION and AMBITION for make your company a success. You want to deliver good quality and safe food products all the time and make a difference compared to others. At Food Safety Experts, we help you to maximise your impact and deliver exceptional results by sharing our knowledge and tools based on industry-wide best practices.

Our belief is that everybody should be able to enjoy safe food at all times. We believe that by sharing our knowledge and tools with QA and Food Safety professionals across the globe, together we will make a difference towards improving food safety for everyone.

OUR VISION

At Food Safety Experts, our vision is a world where safe food is a given for everyone. Our mission is to enable QA and Food Safety professionals to make a difference towards improving food safety. We do this by actively sharing our knowledge and tools and by creating a global community.

For more information, visit
https://www.foodsafety-experts.com